Psychiatry - Theory, Applicatic

Young, Violent and Dangerous to Know

Psychiatry - Theory, Applications, and Treatments

Additional books in this series can be found on Nova's website
under the Series tab.

Additional E-books in this series can be found on Nova's website
under the E-book tab.

PSYCHIATRY - THEORY, APPLICATIONS AND TREATMENTS

YOUNG, VIOLENT AND DANGEROUS TO KNOW

MICHAEL FITZGERALD

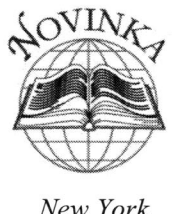

New York

Copyright © 2013 by Nova Science Publishers, Inc.

All rights reserved. No part of this book may be reproduced, stored in a retrieval system or transmitted in any form or by any means: electronic, electrostatic, magnetic, tape, mechanical photocopying, recording or otherwise without the written permission of the Publisher.

For permission to use material from this book please contact us:
Telephone 631-231-7269; Fax 631-231-8175
Web Site: http://www.novapublishers.com

NOTICE TO THE READER

The Publisher has taken reasonable care in the preparation of this book, but makes no expressed or implied warranty of any kind and assumes no responsibility for any errors or omissions. No liability is assumed for incidental or consequential damages in connection with or arising out of information contained in this book. The Publisher shall not be liable for any special, consequential, or exemplary damages resulting, in whole or in part, from the readers' use of, or reliance upon, this material. Any parts of this book based on government reports are so indicated and copyright is claimed for those parts to the extent applicable to compilations of such works.

Independent verification should be sought for any data, advice or recommendations contained in this book. In addition, no responsibility is assumed by the publisher for any injury and/or damage to persons or property arising from any methods, products, instructions, ideas or otherwise contained in this publication.

This publication is designed to provide accurate and authoritative information with regard to the subject matter covered herein. It is sold with the clear understanding that the Publisher is not engaged in rendering legal or any other professional services. If legal or any other expert assistance is required, the services of a competent person should be sought. FROM A DECLARATION OF PARTICIPANTS JOINTLY ADOPTED BY A COMMITTEE OF THE AMERICAN BAR ASSOCIATION AND A COMMITTEE OF PUBLISHERS.

LIBRARY OF CONGRESS CATALOGING-IN-PUBLICATION DATA

Young, violent and dangerous to know / Michael Fitzgerald.
    210 p. ; 26 cm.
Includes bibliographical references and index.
ISBN: 978-1-62257-761-3 (soft cover)
1. Psychopaths. 2.   Antisocial personality disorders.3. Autism. 4. Serial murderers --Mental health. 5. Homicide --psychology. 6.Autistic Disorder --complications. 7. Criminals --psychology. I. Fitzgerald, Michael.
RC555 .F58 2010
      616.85/82

2010001180

Published by Nova Science Publishers, Inc. ✝ New York

Contents

Acknowledgments		vii
Chapter 1	Young, Violent and Dangerous to Know: The Brain of the Serial Killer	1
Chapter 2	Autistic Psychopathy	3
Chapter 3	General Psychopathy and Criminal Autistic Psychopathy	13
Chapter 4	Asperger's Syndrome/Criminal Autistic Psychopathy and Violence	33
Chapter 5	Criminal Autistic Psychopathy and General Psychopathy as a Disorder of Self	41
Chapter 6	Psychological Aspects of (Autistic) Psychopathy	45
Chapter 7	Brain/Psychopathy/Autistic Psychopathy	55
Chapter 8	Evil and Ethics	71
Chapter 9	Dopamine other Neurochemicals, Hormones and Cross Cultural Issues	73
Chapter 10	Serial Killers	83
Chapter 11	Female Serial Killers are Rare	93
Chapter 12	Treatment or Incarceration?	97
Chapter 13	Case Histories of Male Serial Killers and Criminal Autistic Pyscopathy	101
Chapter 14	Case Histories of Female Killers	157
Chapter 15	Conclusion	163
Additional Tables		165
Glossary		169
References		179
Index		197

ACKNOWLEDGMENTS

I wish to thank Therese Carrick, Ellen Cranley and staff of Trinity College Dublin Libarary, Phil Nicholson, Joe O'Brien and Margo Bosonownet, Frances Brennan, Lisa Brennan, Annette Moran, Anne Pritchard, staff of Ballyfermot Child and Family Centre.

Chapter 1

YOUNG, VIOLENT AND DANGEROUS TO KNOW: THE BRAIN OF THE SERIAL KILLER

THE BRAIN, PSYCHOPATHY, CRIMINAL AUTISTIC PSYCHOPATHY AND THE SERIAL KILLER

"Great criminals, as original characters, stand forward on the canvas of humanity as worthy objects of our especial study" (Edmund Burke from The Torture Doctor by David Franke published by Hawthorn Books, New York, 1975).

In Dostoevsky's *Brother Karamazov,* Ivan states that "in every man of course, lies hidden the demon of lustful heat at the screams of the tortured victim, the demon of lawlessness let off the chain".

While murder is a matter of serious concern to the community, serial killing is a matter of even greater concern. Serial killers have baffled the public and professionals for hundreds of years. This book attempts to increase our understanding of serial killers. Fitzgerald (2001, 2003) has suggested that Autistic Psychopathy may underlie some of these serial killers. He suggests a new ddiagnosis Criminal Autistic Psychopathy, which he identifies as a subcategory of Asperger's syndrome. This has had a far greater explanatory power than previously realised. Persons with callous, unemotional traits - often called empathy deficits - are very much associated with Autistic Psychopathy.

Junior civil servants who joined Hitler's killing squads of Jews were multiple killers rather than serial killers. Nevertheless this shows how "normal" human beings could very easily quickly turn in "willing executioners" (Goldhagen, 1997). This is very different from serial killers.

There is only a thin line separating man from barbarity. Nevertheless it is only in the serial killer that we can see the ultimate barbarity and savagery. In "normal' human beings, the brain inhibits these impulses. In some genetically predisposed individuals, the brain, due to faulty neural processes, is unable to do this and hence we have serial killers. There are probably also some environmental inputs, including severe abuse on a genetically predisposed individual in childhood and then a triggering event (e.g. rejection) in later life which can be significant also. Serial killers are in general largely born, but there are still environmental elements which are sometimes labelled "nurture", while the large genetic component is called nature. One of the most prolific serial killers was Gilles de Rais who stated that:

> "I did and perpetrated them (the murders) following the (dictates) of my imagination and my thought, without the advice of anyone, and according to my own judgement and entirely for my own pleasure and physical delight, and for no other intention or end". (Wolf L., 1980)

Wilson quotes from Blake (1971):

> "What is it men in women do require?
> The lineaments of satisfied desire"

Unfortunately in the serial killer, the slow killing of a woman, often including sexual assaults and mutilation of the body, satisfies this desire.

The savagery of the serial killer goes beyond "normal" human comprehension. Dostoevsky in The Brothers Karamazov best describes it:

> "Bestial cruelty, but that's a great injustice to the beast; a beast can never be so cruel as a man, so sadistically cruel. The tiger only tears and gnaws, that's all he can do. He would never think of nailing people by the ears, even if you were able to do it. These Turks took a pleasure in torturing children, too, cutting the unborn child from the mother's womb, and tossing babies up in the air and catching them on the points of their banots before their mother's eyes. Doing it before the mother's eyes was what gave the zest to the amusement" (Dostoevsky in Wolf, 1980).

Tinbergen states that "man is the only species that is a mass murderer . . . the only misfit in his own society" (in Masters (1993).

Wilson (1971) points out that most murders are "crimes of passion". Serial killers do not fit into this category, although they show a tremendous perverse sadistic passion in their slow torturing and killing of their victims. Wilson mentions a murder where the person had "autism" Indeed this is precisely what this book is about and Wilson was very advanced in using this word "autism". Indeed the murderer he describes did possess all the features of autism. Of course it is only a very small subgroup of persons with autism, persons with Criminal Autistic Psychopathy who engage in these acts, less serious aggression though is common.

Serial killers become addicted to killing and need to kill more in order to satisfy their appetite. It is the only thing in life that gives them any satisfaction. This has echoes of Frankenstein. In Robert Louis Stevenson's terms, they become consumed with the nasty Mr. Hyde figure. Simon (1996) is correct to quote Heraclitus who was reported as opining that character is destiny. This fits in with persons with Criminal Autistic Psychopathy. They are born to kill unless they become psychopathic politicians like Hitler, or psychopathic businessmen like Robert Maxwell.

Chapter 2

AUTISTIC PSYCHOPATHY

Criminal Autistic Psychopathy is described in this book as a subtype of Asperger's syndrome and Autism Spectrum Disorders. Lorna Wing first defined Asperger's syndrome in 1981. She used the phrase "Asperger's syndrome' to describe Autistic Psychopathy, which was defined by Hans Asperger in 1944 in Austria. Asperger noted a disturbance in social relationships: "the fundamental disorder of autistic individuals is the limitation of their social relationships. In addition he identified communication difficulties, with abnormalities in the language of autistic individuals. He also identified narrow interests and repetitive activities – "special interests", "abnormal fixations" and "stereotypic movements" He noted associated food fads and unusual reactions to sensory sensations, for example tactile and sound, as well as problems with attention. He was particularly taken with autistic intelligence, but nevertheless stated that the people in question had "all levels of ability from the highly original genius . . . to the . . mentally retarded individual" (Asperger, 1944 and Frith, 1991). Those with reasonable IQ levels portray analytic thinking but poor intuitive thinking. (Wing and Gould, 1979).

Tantum (1991) talks about "people with Asperger's syndrome who make up stories, imaginary words or imaginary play comparisons" They can be massively imaginative (Fitzgerald, 2004) which goes against Lorna Wing and Judith Gould's (1979) emphasis on the impairment of imagination in their triad of impairments in autism.

In 1962, van Krevelen and Kuipers discussed Autistic Psychopathy and emphasised the "personal unapproachability" and the inability "to distinguish between dream and reality" associated with persons with Autistic Psychopathy. They also pointed out that "the eye roams, evades and is turned inwards. The speech is stilted, it is not addressed to the person but into the empty space . . . it sounds false owing to exaggerated inflection".

A similar condition called Autistic Disturbance Of Affective Contact, was described by Leo Kanner in the United States in 1943 as "the profound withdrawal from contact with people, an obsessive desire for the preservation of sameness, a skilful relation to objects, the retention of an intelligent and pensive physiognomy, a kind of language that does not seem intended to serve the purpose of interpersonal communication".

A number of authors have subsequently suggested a number of diagnostic criteria, but the six proposed by Gillberg (1991) are among the most useful descriptions of Asperger's syndrome that I have found:

1. Social impairments.
2. Narrow interests.
3. Repetitive routines.
4. Speech and language peculiarities.
5. Non-verbal communication problems.
6. Motor clumsiness.

Van Krevelen (1962) also emphasises the child's lack of common sense and interest in abstract topics – the "hypertrophy of the intellect at the expense of feeling" The critical factor as Kanner (1943) pointed out is the disturbance of affect.

In 1930, Robert Thorndite described social intelligence as "an ability to perceive their own and others internal states, motivations and behaviour" He also stated that: "Research has validated tests of emotional intelligence and defined it as a set of skills useful in guiding thinking and social interactions" "Emotion was considered irrational by the stoics" Spock of Star Trek (television series) "hailed from the planet Volcan, where pure logic is exalted, making him the consummate Star fleet science officer" Timothy McVeigh, the mass killer, was fascinated by Star Trek.

Salovey and Mayer (2005) also pointed out that "emotion and reason are essentially inseparable". They state that "without feelings, the decisions we make may not be in our best interest" Patients with centromedial prefrontal lesions of the cortex are "unable to use emotion in making decisions". They point out that Damasio stated that "individuals make judgements not only by assessing the severity of outcomes, but also and primarily in terms of their emotional quality". Salovey and Mayer (2005) defined emotional intelligence as "the ability to monitor ones own and others feelings, to discriminate among them, and to use this information to guide ones thinking and action" This is a problem in Criminal Autistic Psychopathy.

SUBTYPING AUTISM SPECTRUM DISORDERS

In relation to autism, Lorna Wing (1998) pointed out that "recognising patterns within this bewildering complexity is akin to classifying clouds".

We must now begin to consider subtyping the Autistic Spectrum Disorder, despite this being an extremely difficult task and various efforts at attempting this have met with failure in the past. Nevertheless, I agree with Luke Tsai (2001), as will be described later, where he made some progress in differentiating autism and Asperger's syndrome. I am hypothesising in this book that selecting Criminal Autistic Psychopathy as a subtype of Asperger's syndrome may stand up or at least to be worthy of future research as a subtype (Fitzgerald 2001; 2003). We miss a great deal by using such a wide category as Autism Spectrum Disorders which blends into normality or using autism as defined by the ADI-R (Lord et al, 1994) which gives an excessively narrow definition of autism.

Autism Spectrum Disorders is too wide an interpretation and "ADI-R autism" is too narrow. Both categories have the effect of limiting research into subtypes. Autism Spectrum Disorder is an enormously heterogeneous condition and to look for one explanation/theory/genetic finding or other neurobiological finding makes no sense.

Subtyping will allow a much increased understanding and greater research potential. The Mind Institute in California is now carrying out an in-depth study of subtyping.

While it is very difficult to make a clear differentiation of autism and Asperger's syndrome (Autistic Psychopathy), I believe they may be at different points on the autistic spectrum, and it may be unwise to dismiss any differences completely. I have some sympathy for the research of Professor Luke Tsai (2001) who noted that the following features were more marked in Asperger's syndrome than in High Functioning Autism:

1. Preoccupation with one or more stereotyped and restricted patterns of interest.
2. Talking, reading and drawing about violence and death.
3. Moody and easily frustrated, with tantrums.
4. Poor hygiene.
5. Failure to develop peer relationships.
6. Interested in heterosexual relationships.
7. Argumentative rules for others.
8. No insight into own disability.
9. Pedantic speech.
10. Likes to tell people his/her special knowledge.

The reader will see that there is support for Luke Tsai's position in relation to some individuals in this book, e.g. an interest in violence by those with Criminal Autistic Psychopathy.

Schultz *et al* (2000) pointed out that there was a tendency to hypothesise about the left hemisphere dysfunction in autism and the right hemisphere dysfunction in Asperger's syndrome. The right hemisphere is normally involved in visuospatial and socio-emotional processing and the left in language, logic, etc. These sharp and consistent differences within Autism and Asperger's syndrome have not been sustained.

In 1979, Hans Asperger in a lecture in England described infantile autism as "highly intelligent children with interesting peculiarities, yet nevertheless with behaviour so difficult that they were almost impossible to keep in family or school. They achieve the highest university professorships or become artists – yet their quirks and peculiarities will remain with them for life" This book is about the quirks and peculiarities of those with Criminal Autistic Psychopathy. For differential diagnosis, see **Table 1**.

Hans Asperger (1979) stated that "it has become obvious that the conditions described by myself and Leo Kanner concern basically different types, yet in some respects there is complete agreement", and that his "typical cases are very intelligent children with extraordinary originality of thought and spontaneity of activity though their actions are not always the right response to the prevailing situation" These inappropriate responses of people are described in this book. Asperger (1974) also states that:

Table 1A. Differential Diagnosis of Criminal Autistic Psychopathy

Criminal Autistic Psychopathy	Impairment in use of eye-to-eye gaze, facial expression, body postures	Failure to develop peer relationships to developmental level	Lack of spontaneous seeking to share enjoyment	Lack of social and emotional reciprocity	Preoccupation with one or more stereotyped patterns of interest	Inflexible adherence to specific non-functional routines or rituals
Autistic psychopathy						
Schizoid personalty in childhood		Yes.	Yes.	Yes.	Yes.	Yes.
Semantic pragmatic disorder		Yes.	Yes, sometimes.	Yes.		
Narcissistic Personality Disorder		Yes, sometimes.	Yes.	Yes.		Yes.
Non-verbal learning Disability		Yes.		Yes.		
Schizotypal disorder		Yes.	Yes.	Yes.	Yes, sometimes.	
Attention deficit hyperactivity disorder		Yes, sometimes.		Yes, often.		
Schizophrenia	Yes.		Yes.	Yes.		
Autistic-like disorders	Yes.	Yes.	Yes.	Yes.	Yes.	Yes.
General psychopathy	Yes, sometimes.	Yes.	Yes.	Yes.	Yes, sometimes.	

Table 1B. Differential Diagnosis of Criminal Autistic Psychopathy

Criminal Autistic Psychopathy	Stereotyped and repetitive motor mannerism	Persistent preoccupation with parts of objects	Clinically significant impairment in social or occupational functioning	No clinically significant delay in language development	No clinically significant delay in cognitive development or self-help skills
Autistic psychopathy					
Schizoid personalty in childhood			Yes.	Yes.	Yes.
Semantic pragmatic disorder			Yes.		Yes.
Narcissistic Personality Disorder			Yes, sometimes	Yes.	Yes.
Non-verbal learning dsability			Yes.		
Schizotypal disorder			Yes.	Yes.	Yes.
Attention deficit hyperactivity disorder			Yes.	Yes.	Yes.
Schizophrenia	Yes, sometimes catatonic.		Yes.	Disorganised speech can be evident.	
Autistic-like disorders			Yes.		
General psychopathy			Yes.	Formally called Semantic Aphasia. Often no.	Often no.

"their thinking, too, seems unusual in that it is endowed with special abilities in the areas of logic and abstraction and these often follow their own cause with no regard for outside influences. Often they are not directed towards the wider world, but are canalised into rather abstruse subjects of little practical use A further important difference from early infantile autism is that Asperger children, very early, even before they walk, develop highly grammatical speech and they may be uncommonly apt at using expressions coined spontaneously. There is a likeness here to children described by Kanner (1943). However, the children with Kanner's syndrome generally avoid communication, and they do not develop speech or else develop it very late. But even autistic children with the Asperger's syndrome who have complete speech, do not usually use it for communication. It seems that they do not wish to convey information to others or do not want to get into contact with them; rather they hold forth on their own subject of interest and do not appear to care whether others wish to listen or whether they are speaking out of turn."

They show evidence of autistic narrative that is problems with the practical aspects of language and often speak in monologues.

As far as this book is concerned, their interests can be very dangerous, e.g. violence and serial killing.

Mesibov (2001) and colleagues note points made by Bosch that "remain relevant today."

"In describing Autistic Psychopathy, Bosch asserts that the difference between Asperger's syndrome and autism is a matter of degree, and that the same person can be diagnosed with each disorder at different points in life. Bosch asserts that many people with Asperger's syndrome (Autistic Psychopathy) would have been diagnosed with autism if they had been seen at younger ages. Likewise some of his patients with autism improved enough with age to be indistinguishable from his adult clients with Asperger's syndrome (Autistic Psychopathy). The possibility of different diagnosis at different ages is still discussed today."

A differentiation was made in DSM-IV (APA, 2000) between autism and Asperger's syndrome although it was done in a very confused way by demanding no clinically significant general delay in language. In reality, language problems are very common in Asperger's syndrome.

The differentiation between autism and Asperger's syndrome has been well discussed by Kugler (1998), who states that "few definitive conclusions can be drawn".

Wing (1991) notes that Kanner stated that: "it is well known in medicine that any illness may appear in different degrees of severity, all the way from so-called formes frustes to the most fulminant manifestations. Does this possibly apply also to . . . autism?". The answer is "yes". This book demonstrates a fulminant form – Criminal Autistic Psychopathy.

Hans Asperger stated that "it was the astonishing similarities within these two groups (autism/Asperger's syndrome) which obviously accounted for the same choice of name. The two types are at once so alike and yet so different. When Kanner writes of an innate phenomenon of a peculiar disability to form affective contacts, then this is just as valid for the Asperger type. And all those who have tried to interpret the nature of the disturbance have made similar statements. We, in this country, speak of a defect in the "thymic", the mind of the personality. This defect would explain the disturbance in relationship to other people and of all that builds up human contact" This defect is critical to Autistic Psychopathy which was seen as a personality disorder by Hans Asperger. This idea has been revived in this book.

Uta Frith (1991), carried out a magnificent translation of Hans Asperger's (1944) work pointing out that Autistic Psychopathy could also be called "Autistic Personality Disorder". With new developments in neurobiology I would be happy with either diagnostic classification.

Lorna Wing prefers to call Asperger's syndrome a developmental disorder and disagreed with classifying "Asperger's syndrome as a personality disorder instead of viewing it as a developmental problem on the Autism Spectrum" (Wing, 1986). Lorna Wing always pushed for a broader conceptualisation of autism that is the broader autism phenotype many years before this was accepted. Many researchers at the same time were demanding that autism be described as a narrow condition using only Kanner's narrow criteria. This was extremely damaging and prevented huge numbers of patients on the Autism Spectrum from getting the treatment that they deserved. Happily this narrow conceptualisation of autism has been now been abandoned. Wing dislike of Autistic Psychopathy was because it was associated with Antisocial Personality. I am now arguing for the opposite that there is a subcategory of Asperger's syndrome, as Wing defined it, who would be much better described by Hans Asperger's phrase Autistic Psychopathy or as Criminal Autistic Psychopathy the term I use in this book.

Kendell (2002) makes the point that I fully agree with, that "the historical reasons for regarding personality disorders as fundamentally different from mental illnesses are being undermined by both clinical and genetic evidence".

In actual fact, I believe that Hans Asperger was not incorrect when he described Autistic Psychopathy as a personality disorder in his initial paper. The distinction between a developmental disorder like Autistic Psychopathy and a personality disorder has become increasingly blurred with genetic and biological underpinnings to both.

Kurt Schneider (1950) described personality disorders as "abnormal varieties of sane psychic life" and this would fit with Criminal Autistic Psychopathy with diminished responsibility and odd behaviour.

Personality types and developmental disorders like Asperger's syndrome can be seen as representing extremes of normal variation, with the exception of Criminal Autistic Psychopathy which I see as a category. I view these conditions as biomedical phenomena. Clearly there are many pejorative value judgments associated with personality disorders. Scadding (1967) used the term "biological disadvantage" and this is a term which I am very much at ease with and find very useful.

Of course as I have shown in my book, *Autism and Creativity* (2004), biological disadvantage in one area is often associated with creativity or advantage in another area. Kendell (2002) is correct to point out that "it is becoming increasing clear that the genetic bases of affective personality disorders and mood disorders, and of Schizoid Personality Disorder and schizophrenia, have much in common". I would add Asperger's syndrome/Criminal Autistic Psychopathy subtype to this.

Pilgrim (2002) notes that Kendell "a psychiatrist, also argues that a dimensional view makes more sense (he calls them "greater traits") – suggesting that a categorical approach has now failed us all, both scientifically and pragmatically". This is precisely my view with a few exceptions.

One can see that many features of Autistic Psychopathy are contained in many of the personality disorder diagnosis of DSM-IV and ICD10. These would include a detachment from social relations, a restricted range of emotional expression, suspiciousness, problems with interpersonal relationships and self image, discomfort in close relationships, hypersensitivity to negative evaluation, disregard for violation of the rights of others, grandiosity, and lack of empathy.

It is easy to see why Criminal Autistic Psychopathy would not be diagnosed and that other diagnoses would be given instead for example Schizoid, Paranoid, Borderline, Schizotypal, Avoidant, Compulsive, Antisocial or Narcissistic Personality Disorder. In terms of the odd cluster of cognitive-perceptual organisation, Dolan and Millington (2004) put in here Schizotypal, Schizoid and Paranoid Personality Disorders. They note that this odd cluster has "unusual or paranoid ideas, social isolation, and odd styles of interacting with the environment. They are frequently also characterised by an inability to establish and maintain interpersonal relationships" All these features are features of Criminal Autistic Psychopathy.

The overlap can further be seen in Dolan and Millington's (2004) description of persons with schizoid psychopathology as having a detachment from social relations and restricted range of emotional expression. The person with paranoid psychopathology is described as being distrustful and suspicious and you get this in Autistic Psychopathy. The person with a borderline psychopathology is described as having an instability in interpersonal relationships, instability in self-image, instability in affects, and being impulsive - all features which can occur in Autistic Psychopathy. The person with Schizotypal psychopathology is described as having acute discomfort in close relationships, in having cognitive or perceptual distortions and eccentricities of behaviour all of which can occur in Autistic Psychopathy. The person with avoidant personality has social inhibitions, feelings of inadequacy and hypersensitivity to negative evaluation - all of which can occur in Autistic Psychopathy. Fitzgerald (2005) emphasises the overlap between Borderline Personality Disorder and Asperger's syndrome. Those with compulsive psychopathology are described as having a preoccupation with orderliness, perfectionism and control -all of which can occur in Autistic Psychopathy. The person with antisocial psychopathology has a disregard for and violates the rights of others, and the person with narcissistic psychopathology has a grandiosity, lack of empathy, all of which can occur in Autistic Psychopathy. The reason that personality disorder has not been described much in childhood appears to be due to political correctness and the feeling that to apply one of these personality disorders to children is unduly negative and pessimistic. I disagree with this. Clearly a dimensional approach to diagnosis is necessary as well as putting people on multiple dimensions.

Dolan and Millington (2004) also point out something that is critical, and is my view, that in childhood and in adulthood there is some degree of overlap in the presentation of individuals who suffer from personality disorders within this cluster and those who suffer on the extreme of social withdrawal dimension what I would call Autistic Psychopathy. While there is some debate as to whether schizoid and Schizotypal Personality Disorders are pervasive developmental disorders, Wolff (1995) recommends that in "children who do not manifest gross impairment, a personality disorder diagnosis may be more appropriate".

Autistic Psychopathy is sometimes confused with Multiple Personality Disorder. This is because people with Autistic Psychopathy have identity diffusion, multiple selves, Jekyll and Hyde figures where the Hyde figure become dominant as time goes on. Another error in the DSM-III diagnosis (1980) was to have a category of Multiple Personality Disorder as a stress induced disorder. The DSM-IV (APA, 1994) is now changed to Dissociated Identity Disorder. Autistic Psychopathy should be considered as a differential diagnosis of that category.

SENSORY PROBLEMS IN AUTISTIC PSYCHOPATHY

Bogdashina (2005) notes that in relation to Temple Grandin's 1996 work that "there is a continuum of sensory processing problems for most autistic people, which goes from fractured disjoined images at one end to a slight abnormality at the other cornerstone of autism" Some of the persons with Criminal Autistic Psychopathy are hypersensitive to noise. She points out that autism "is about sensory differences which is far more complicated than, for example, tactile defensiveness". She also points out that "not all differences in perception are dysfunctional". She notes that "some may be interpreted as strengths or even super abilities that can become dysfunctional if not recognised by the outside world. No one can guess that their eyes, for example, pick up different signals form the light, shade, colour and movement". Here she is referring to Blackman (2001).

Persons with autism according to Bogdashina "are often unaware that they perceive the world differently from the other 99% of the population, because they have nothing to compare their perception with. The first realisation of their differences usually comes in the late teens or even later". They can blame themselves for their problems. Bogdashina also states that "unselected information cannot be processed simultaneously and may lead to sensory information overload" Persons with Criminal Autistic Psychopathy can show this. There can also be delayed mental processing. As usual you can have hypersensitivity or hyposensitivity again evidence of the heterogeneity of autism. She discusses monoprocessing which she says is an effort "to limit the amount of information and avoid distortions, fragmentation and overload, autistic people may use one sensory channel at a time, while the rest of the senses are on hold. It brings certain restriction to their perception but helps them to make sense of information in at least one sensory modality" When they are overwhelmed with sensory stimuli they can withdraw, be unresponsive to questioning, and appear 'deaf' They have a very narrow focus which also decreases sensory inputs. Problems with set shifting (moving from one area of attention to another) also reduces sensory inputs.

Interests

Persons with Autistic Psychopathy tend to have their own interests and are experimentalists for example in the areas of chemistry and poisons. They can design unique experiments. They are often interested in nature, animals, and the insides of animals and human beings. This can feature in the serial killing of persons with Criminal Autistic Psychopathy. They are extremely bored by the activities of children in the schoolyard and are therefore often excluded and bullied. They love dismantling mechanical objects and often become engineers, inventors, computer specialists, mechanics and electricians. They tend to be massive readers and prefer the company of books to human beings.

Control

Persons with Autistic Psychopathy are extremely controlling. Ogden (1989) points out that "pathological autism aims at the absolute elimination of the unknown and the unpredictable". This is what Dahlmer did in his serial killing. This eliminated the unpredictable behaviour of humans (Ogden 1989). He also points out that "the machine like predictability of experiences with pathological autistic shapes and objects substitutes for experiences with inevitably imperfect and not entirely predictable human beings. No person can compete with the capacity of never-changing autistic shapes and objects to provide absolutely reliable comfort and protection". This has echoes of Dahlmer who believed that when his victims were dead or unconscious they were predicable and under his power and control.

Prevalence of Autism/Asperger's Syndrome

The National Autistic Society (2001) in the United Kingdom estimated the possible total prevalence rate of all autistic spectrum disorders at 91 per 100,000 broken down as follows:

1. People with learning disability with an IQ under 70:
   (a) Classic autism, 5 per 10,000 (McCarthy, Fitzgerald & Smith (1984) found a rate of autism of 4.3 per 10,000).
   (b) Other spectrum disorders, 15 per 10,000.
2. People with average or high ability:
   (a) Asperger's syndrome / High Functioning Autism, 36 per 10,000.
   (b) Other spectrum disorders, 35 per 10,000.

Fombonne (2005) estimated the arte of Asperger's syndrome at "4.3 per 10,000" which would be considered a low figure. Eric Fombonne (2005) states that "taking 35 per 10,000 to 60 per 10,000 as two working rates for the combination of all Pervasive Developmental Disorders and using US population figures as of July 1, 2002, it can be estimated that about 248,000 and up to 486,000 subjects under the age of 20 years suffer from Pervasive Developmental Disorder in the United States".

In terms of prevalence of autism, the Office of National Statistics (ONS) found the prevalence of autism in 5 to 15 year olds at 1%. I agree with the estimate of about 1% for all Autism Spectrum Disorders.

> "Autism which affects as many as 1.5 million people is currently the fastest growing developmental disability in America" (Looking Up, 2005).

Posserud *et al* (2006), found in a total population study using the Autism Spectrum Screening Questionnaire completed by children and parents, a rate of 2.1% high scorers. This may contain those who would in future be misdiagnosed as having General Psychopathy.

The "estimate" prevalence in the UK could put the figure of Autism Spectrum Disorder at close to a half million. The individuals discussed in this book are the kind of people who have been missed in the past and there is serious under diagnosis of Asperger's syndrome and atypical autism throughout the world, particularity in Forensic populations.

Pervasive Developmental Disorders is an overarching category which includes Autistic disorders, Pervasive Developmental Disorder Not Otherwise Specified, Rett's Disorder, Childhood Disintegrative Disorder, and Asperger's Syndrome.

Chapter 3

GENERAL PSYCHOPATHY AND CRIMINAL AUTISTIC PSYCHOPATHY

Schreiber wrote about a murderer in "*The Shoemaker*" This murderer stated, "I had a lack of feeling that I was a part of anybody – or that anybody was a part of me". (Flora Rheta Schreiber, 1983).

DEFINITION

The *Oxford Companion to the Mind* (2004) states that psychopathy is the "inability to tolerate minor frustration, an incapacity for forming stable emotional relationships, a failure to learn from past experience . . and a tendency to act impulsively or recklessly". The *Oxford Companion* goes on to further describe three kinds of psychopathy "predominantly inadequate, the predominantly aggressive, and the creative psychopath" My view is that the composer Richard Wagner was a creative Autistic Psychopath. Psychopaths who come from rich families may turn out to be psychopathic businessmen or psychopathic politicians, and may not come to criminal attention and indeed are often admired.

Schneider (1958) described "psychopathic" personalities as being associated with a "marked emotional blunting mainly but not exclusively in relation to their fellows. Their character is a pitiless one and they lack the capacity for shame, decency, remorse, and conscience. They are ungracious, cold, surly, and brutal in crime, . . . the moral code is known, understood but not felt and therefore [this] personality is indifferent to it" Many of these features also occur in those with Criminal Autistic Psychopathy. They are sometimes diagnosed as having Schizoid Psychopathy.

Pinel (1801) noted that these persons were "marked by abstract and sanguinary fury, with a blind propensity to acts of violence".

Kraepelin (1909 – 1915) used the word psychopathic to include all abnormal personalities. He did have an eccentric subtype and a type called unrepentant which fits in with the current concepts of psychopathic personality. The eccentric subtype fits particularly well with Criminal Autistic Psychopathy.

In *Clinical Psychiatry,* Slater Roth (1969) wrote that: "the social legal importance of the emotionally callous psychopath is considerable . . . this quality of personality contributes to the makeup of societies most ruthless, dangerous and incorrigible criminals. However, it must not be assumed that the emotionally callous are invariably criminal . . . their lack of capacity for human feeling and their lack of need for the affection, the friendship and the understanding of others, is like a blind spot of personality". They also point out that the callous psychopath will have been found to be "generally unresponsive, incapable of friendship, or even of a natural affection to his parents. For reasons, into which genetical and environmental causes may both enter, his parents have frequently shown some of the same traits too" Parents of persons with Criminal Autistic Psychopathy often show similar traits.

Persons with Psychopathy have very high rates of recidivism. They are Jekyll and Hyde figures. Clekley (1976) saw psychopathic violence as instrumental. By that I mean it was less likely to be reactive. The various backgrounds to violence that are discussed in this book are: (1) instrumental which is more volitional, and (2) reactive.

PREVALENCE

Blair *et al* (2005) estimated that there are "psychopathic tendencies of between 1.23% and 3.46% i.e. approximately one quarter of the incidence rate of Conduct Disorder in community samples". Up to a quarter of all persons in US prisons would meet the criteria for psychopathy. At least twice as many males as females meet the psychopathy criteria.

PSYCHOPATHIC TRAITS IN CHILDHOOD

According to Sonderstrom (2003), psychopathy is a personality disorder with "childhood onset sharing common clinical dysfunctions with Attention Deficit Hyperactivity Disorder and Autism Spectrum Disorders" and is "an empathy disorder characterised by mentalising problems, poor coherence, emotional disturbances, social brain dysfunction, and poor character maturation". I fully agree with this statement and indeed this is a central theme of my book.

Viding *et al* (2005) in a twin study of psychopathic tendencies in young children, showed that those with high levels of callous unemotional traits showed "extremely strong genetic influence" and "no influence of shared environment".

Hill (2002) notes that "callous unemotional traits . . . are central to psychopathy in childhood just as they are in adult life". Fitzgerald (2003) emphasised these callous unemotional traits in Asperger's syndrome. Golding's novel *Lord of the Flies* -about sadistic behaviour in boys - is probably more in the domain of secondary psychopathy where environmental factors are critical.

Diagnostic and Statistical Manual (American Psychiatric Association, 1968, 1980, 1987, 1994) and Psychopathy

DSM-II (1968) used the term sociopath instead of psychopath. DSM-II also describes the so-called sociopath as selfish, callous, irresponsible, impulsive person who lacks a capacity to learn from experience, blames others for their problems, and showed poor frustration tolerance.

Stone (1993) points out that the word sociopath means that "something is wrong with one's actions in society" while psychopath means that "there was something wrong with one's mind" There was no need to change psychopath to sociopath. This was a serious error influenced by sociology, socio-babble, and a social psychiatry that had lost its way. Nevertheless there are environmental factors present in psychopathy. If sociopathy applies at all, it applies to the secondary psychopath.

ICD10 (WHO, 1992) states that personality disorders "represent either extreme or significant deviations from the way the average individual perceives, thinks, feels, and particularly relates to others'. This fits in precisely with Asperger's syndrome or Autistic Psychopathy. Criminal Autistic Psychopathy is qualitatively different in terms of its extreme behaviour or manifestation.

PRIMARY AND SECONDARY PSYCHOPATHY

Primary psychopathy (which overlaps with Criminal Autistic Psychopathy) is largely genetic, while secondary psychopathy has a significant environmental component or indeed a largely environmental component with genetic factors being much less signifcant than with primary psychopathy. A high IQ does not protect the psychopath from serial killing if they are that way inclined.

Persons with Psychopathy show poor fear conditioning. They live very much in the present time. They think little about the future and are mainly preoccupied about getting satisfaction in the present. Again here there is an overlap between General Psychopathy and Criminal Autistic Psychopathy.

Persons with Psychopathy have extreme emotional deficits and a lack of capacity to interact on a normal social emotional level. They tend to be rather fearless. The same could be said of Criminal Autistic Psychopathy - a subgroup of Asperger's syndrome. There is a broad spectrum of psychopathy, which includes Criminal Autistic Psychopathy. Criminal Autistic Psychopaths can show autistic charm which can impress people and they can be described as witty as Ludwig Wittgenstein who had Autistic Psychopathy was described. A capacity for humour can be present (Lyons and Fitzgerald, 2004).

Variability and heterogeneity in the clinical picture is normal in presentation. Persons with psychopathy can be cunning and cold in personality. They lack a depth of care for people, a lack of respect for human beings who are only seen as being there to fulfil their needs. They lack the capacity to put themselves in other people's shoes from an emotional point of view. They can be extremely persuasive and because they have a very narrow focus and put all their energy at times into this focus, this can lead to them being very successful and being able to con people. They want society to adapt to them rather than them adapting to society. When one reads about psychopathy and (Lykken, 2006) Psychopathic Personality, one could easily mistake Lykken's descriptions for Autistic Psychopathy, although Asperger's syndrome and Autistic Psychopathy are not used in this current 2006 definitive *Handbook on Psychopathy* Lykken (2006) emphasises the socio-emotional problems, the impulsivity, the fearlessness, and the temper tantrums persons with psychopathy have as children. He also emphasises the genetic component. The same could be said of Criminal Autistic Psychopathy.

Clearly Criminal Autistic Psychopathy or any form of psychopathy is not a totally genetic phenomenon, as there are also environmental elements. One might speculate that if people with this genetic predisposition have an excellent caring, warm and supportive family environment, they might turn out to be so called successful psychopaths in politics or business rather than criminal psychopaths e.g. Sir Richard Burton and Lyndon Johnson. (Patrick, 2006).

Levin and Fox (1985) provided a good description of psychopathy when they wrote that "they are not sick in either a medical or legal sense. Instead the serial killer is typically a sociopathic personality who lacks, internal controls – guilt or conscience – to guide his own behaviour, but has excessive need to control and dominate others. He definitely knows right from wrong, definitely realises he has committed a sinful act, but simply doesn't care about his human prey. The sociopath has never internalised a moral code that prohibits murder. Having fun is all that counts".

Blair *et al* (2006) state that psychopathy involves "a pattern of both emotional (considerably reduced empathy and guilt) and behavioural (criminal activity and, frequently, violence) symptoms. We argue that the emotional component is the crucial component of psychopathy. There are many developmental routes to an elevated risk for antisocial behaviour. The emotional dysfunction that is at the heart of psychopathy is only one such route. However, it is one that puts the individual at heightened risk for learning antisocial behaviours. Although, as will be argued, it does not necessarily mean that the individual will learn to be antisocial; whether he / she does or not will be determined by a constellation of individual and social factors".

Dostoevsky had Versilov state in one of his novels "I am split mentally . . . . It is as if you have your own double standing next to you". Brian Masters (1993) points out that there is a similar theme in James Hogg's book *The Private Memoirs and Confessions of a Justified Sinner*.

Albert Camus wrote about such a character called Meursault in *The Stranger*. This is about a man who got involved in a mindless detached killing – psychopathic killing. Psychological splitting is a feature of these conditions.

Karpmin (1948) pointed out that "the primary psychopath often acts purposefully and directly to maximise his gain or excitement, whereas the secondary psychopath typically acts out of such emotions as hatred and revenge, often in reaction to circumstances that exacerbate his or her neurotic conflict".

The primary psychopath overlaps with Criminal Autistic Psychopathy. According to Karpmin (1941), fearlessness was associated with primary psychopathy but not secondary psychopathy. The primary psychopath is more likely to plan their criminal activities, while the secondary psychopath is more likely to react to environmental stresses. Kalman's 1938 so-called "Schizoid Psychopaths" would fit in with Criminal Autistic Psychopathy and primary psychopathy. It is likely that secondary psychopathy could emerge from severe sexual abuse or gross deprivation, or neglect in childhood.

According to Karpmin (1948) the true primary psychopath "is in a sense the least impulsive of them all . . Rather than being hasty, the psychopath often coolly and deliberately plans his action . . there is no hot headedness here at all of the type we are accustomed to seeing in neurotics and psychotics" Persons with Criminal Autistic Psychopathy often plan their actions.

Mealy (1995) states that "primary sociopaths", are individuals of a certain genotype, phenotype, and personality who are incapable of experiencing the secondary "social" emotions that normally contribute to behavioural motivation and inhibition. The same can be said about Criminal Autistic Psychopathy.

Blair *et al* (2006) point out that "abuse is unlikely to lead to the affective 'flattening' that is core feature of psychopathy". They also state that "however, we do not believe, on the basis of the available data, that physical/sexual abuse is a key factor in the genesis of psychopathy." A defining feature of psychopathy is the reduction, not elevation, in the individual's responsiveness to threat (Clekley, 1976; Hare, 1970; Lykken, 1995; Patrick, 1994). Indeed, it is even possible that the neurobiological basis of psychopathy may protect the individual with psychopathic tendencies from developing mood and anxiety disorders such as depression, anxiety and Post Traumatic Stress Disorder". In the real clinical world, the picture is much more mixed. But Criminal Autistic Psychopathy may fit in with Blair *et al*'s (2006) view.

Blair *et al*'s (2006) view probably applies to primary psychopaths. Nevertheless, I believe that genetic and environmental factors are cumulative in primary psychopathy with a much greater emphasis on the genetic factors. While persons with primary psychopathy have less affective symptoms, I do not believe that these are absent as some of the cases in this book show. While persons with Autistic Psychopathy show a great deal of affective symptoms, persons with the Criminal Autistic Psychopathy subtype show very little, again showing the overlap with primary psychopathy.

Characteristics of psychopathy have been defined by a number of authors Clekley (1941, 1967 and, Hare (1991) as:

- A lack of empathy,
- A lack of guilt,
- an empathy deficits,
- shallow affect,
- callous behaviour,
- easily bored, and
- impulsive behaviour.

They also tend to ignore social norms and values and show inappropriate reactions when challenged about their behaviour as do persons with Criminal Autistic Psychopathy. (Clekley, 1941, Cooke and Michie 2001) point out that "there is compelling evidence for psychopathy's utility" and that "it is an important prediction of criminal behaviour, particularly violence" and is also linked to "failure on conditional release, violent recidivism" Cooke and Michie (2001) noted personality traits in psychopathy as being – "emotional coldness, incapacity for love, egocentricity, fearlessness, and absence of anxiety". These are also seen in Autistic Psychopathy (Fitzgerald, 2001).

Psychopathy is a personality construct and there is evidence for its coherence. Cooke and Michie, *et al* (2005) showed that the "syndromal structure of psychopathy was invariant across cultures". I believe the same can be said about Criminal Autistic Psychopathy.

Psychopathic Novelty Seeking and Sensation Seeking

In Harper et al's (1989) two-factor model of psychopathy, they include very important items such as the need for stimulation and proneness to boredom. There is some evidence that novelty seeking is linked to polymorphisms in the dopamine genes (DRD4) (Holmes et al, 2002; Kirley et al, 2004; Lowe et al, 2004). These are often associated with Attention Deficit Hyperactivity Disorder, which is not an uncommon precursor of psychopathy. Novelty seeking is a critical component of the psychopathy concept. (Harpur et al, 1989).

According to Millon et al, Cloninger (1987) regards the primary psychopath "as being high in novelty seeking, low in the desire to avoid harm, and low dependence on external rewards".

Vallone et al (2000) point out that DRD4 (Dopamine D4 Receptor) is expressed in the frontal cortex, amygdala and hippocampus.

Links have been shown between DRD4 polymorphism and novelty seeking. According to Laucht et al (2005), Cloninger et al (1993) conceptualised novelty seeking as a "dopaminergic modulated and heritable tendency towards excitement in response to" specific excitatory stimuli. In relation to this book it would be identifying a suitable victim for sexual, sadistic serial killing.

I have also noticed clinically novelty seeking prevalent in Asperger's syndrome, which I call Autistic Novelty Seeking. I believe there is a considerable overlap between Attention Deficit Hyperactivity Disorder and Autism (Fitzgerald et al, 2006).

Plomin et al (2004) also note the hypothesis "that there is a reward mechanism whereby novelty seeking promotes dopamine release, and that individuals with less efficient long-repeat DRD4 allele have to "work harder" to seek novelty and increase dopamine release". Killing must be the ultimate stimulus. It is possible that this is the neurochemical mechanism by which serial killers get their buzz or thrill. They take more risks to get the same buzz as their killing careers progress.

Borderline Personality Disorder (BPD)

Borderline Personality Disorder can be confused with Criminal Autistic Psychopathy. Anthony Ryle (1997) has a model of Borderline Personality Disorder, which he describes as "multiple self states model". It is hardly surprising that Asperger's syndrome and Borderline Personality Disorder could be confused, because this concept of a multiple self states model is equally applicable to Asperger's syndrome/Autistic Psychopathy and Criminal Autistic Psychopathy. I describe it as identity diffusion. (Ryle, 1997, Fitzgerald, 2001, 2004, 2005).

Dietz (1986) argues against diagnostically labelling of these men as Borderline Personality Disorders, emphasising that "these men may enjoy killing people". They do not have Borderline Personality Disorder, but they do have Criminal Autistic Psychopathy or General Psychopathy.

Indeed, Blackburn (1996) regards secondary psychopaths as "predominantly borderline personalities". This makes sense as secondary psychopathy have a greater environmental input into aetiology.

Sadistic Personality Disorder (SPD)

Sadistic Personality Disorder was discussed in DSM-III-R (APA, 1987). It is a form of psychopathy. SPDs are characterised by criteria which include using violence to establish dominance, humiliating people, taking pleasure in other peoples' suffering, and threatening others.

Spitzer *et al* (1991) discuss the proposed diagnostic criteria for Sadistic Personality Disorder in DSM-III-R. In my view, many of the features could fit with Criminal Autistic Psychopathy, including using "physical cruelty or violence for the purpose of establishing dominance". Other features include showing a lack of empathy by demeaning persons in the presence of others, being extremely unempathetic and overly critical in dealing with subordinates, taking pleasure in physical cruelty to animals, intimidating people, over controlling people, and being fascinated by weapons of aggression including guns etc.

Antisocial Personality Disorder (APA, DSM-IV 1994) (ASPD)

In the *Handbook of Psychopathy*, (Patrick, eds, 2006) is stated that *Psychopathy and DSM-IV psychopathology (*Widiger) points out that "the description of APD (Antisocial Personality Disorder) within the 2nd Edition of the American Psychiatric Association 1968 DSM resembles reasonably well the description of psychopathy provided by Clekley in 1941" Widiger (2006) points out that "many studies have indicated that the construct of psychopathy has been successful in identifying a particularly callous, dangerous, and remorseless subset of criminals who repeatedly engage in particular heinous, brutal, and exploitive acts. Psychopathic persons begin their criminal careers earlier, commit a greater variety of offences, and offend at higher rates"

ASPD (Antisocial Personality Disorder) is characterised by a failure to conform to social norms, deceitfulness, impulsivity, aggressiveness, a reckless disregard for the safety of self or others, consistent irresponsible disability, and lack of remorse. This is less severe than psychopathy but is on a spectrum with it.

Blair *et al* (2005) in examining Antisocial Personality Disorder and Psychopathy state that "it is not that psychopathy extends the DSM-IV diagnosis (ASPD) because it considers personality, but rather that it extends these diagnoses because it considers emotion".

The similarities and differences between HFA/ASP and Antisocial Personality Disorder are shown in **Table 3**.

McDonald and Iacono, 2006) state that "Psychopathy overlaps with but is not the same as, anti-sociality, yet much of the etiologically relevant research deals broadly with antisocial behaviour".

The diagnosis of Antisocial Personality Disorder simply does not cover psychopathy in a meaningful way. It is the severity of the callous-unemotional traits that converts Antisocial Personality Disorder or Conduct Disorder in childhood into psychopathy. Callous – unemotional traits predict a persistence in offending. Fitzgerald (2003) has noted these unemotional traits in Asperger's syndrome. Fitzgerald. (2003).

Table 3A. Similarities and Differences between HFA/ASP and Antisocial personality

Antisocial personality/psychopathy	Autistic Personality
Super ego deficits.	Harsh superego.
Morality reduced.	Morality generally increased, but with very serious exceptions due to lack of capacity for empathy.
Serotonin (low tendency).	Serotonin (high tendency).
Primary psychopaths have 'semantic aphasis' This was first described by Checky in 1951.(Millon and Davis, 2000) Semantic aphasis refers to 'meaning, and aphasis is broadly considers a class of disorders related to the understanding or production of language... Psychopaths suffer an inborn inability to understand and express meaning of emotional experience, even though their understanding of meaning is normal.'	Difficulties in semantic pragmatic problems are very important in HFA/ASP, as are problems in understanding the meaning of experience.
'The significance of embarrassment [and] shame is lost on them'.	Same features as in autistic psychopathy.
Problems in understanding 'what makes people tick.'	Same.
Problems in adapting to 'the alien world of the empathic and socialised.'	Same.
'unable to apprise a potentially dangerous situation by gauging their own fear, they plough ahead violently, regardless of risk.'	This can occur in autistic psychopathy.
'Low in the desire to avoid harm, and low in dependence on external awards.'	This can occur in autistic psychopathy with violent propensities.
Heredity element	Higher heredity element.
DSM-IV antisocial personality disorder (American Psychiatric Association, 1994): 1. Persuasive patterns of disregard for and violation of the right of others occurring since age of 15 years. 2. Failure to conform to social norms. 3. Deceitfulness. 4. Impulsivity. 5. Irritability and agressivity. 6. Disregard for the safety of self and others. 7. Repeated failure to maintain consistent work behaviour. 8. Lack of remorse.	1. Autistic psychopathy occurs before and after 15 years. 2. Occurs in autistic psychopathy. 3. Does not occur in autistic psychopathy. 4. Common in autistic psychopathy. 5. Not uncommon in autistic psychopathy. 6. Can occur in autistic psychopathy. 7. Common in autistic psychopathy 8. Common in autistic psychopathy.
Illness model is inappropriate for the concept of psychopathy. (Dolan & Coid, 1993).	Same.
Persons who are given the diagnosis are not a homogenous group. (Gunn in Gaind, 1978).	Same.
Could be a final common pathway for a series of different conditions. (Dolan & Coid, 1993).	Same.

Table 3B.

Brian problems	Criminal Autistic Psychopathy	General Psychopathy
Frontal lobe.	Abnormalities.	Reduced glucose metabolism (murders). Reduced grey matter.
Posterior hippocampus.		Reduced volume.
Amygdala.	Abnormalities small in adults.	Reduced volume and malfunctioning.
Corpus callosum.	? Reduced.	Enlarged.
Cerebellum.	Abnormal.	
Bain white matter.	White matter increase.	White matter increased in liars.
Brian grey matter.		Reduced grey matter.
Problems fusiform face area of brain.	Yes, problems.	? Yes.
Von Economo Neurons	Yes problems	? Yes.
Minicolumns	Yes problems	? Yes.
Autonomic nervous system	? Reduced activity in Criminal Autistic Psychopathy, increased in non-criminal autism.	Reduced activity.
Insula.		Malfunctioning.
Temporal lobe.		Abnormalities.
Cerebral lateralisation.	Variable.	Less lateralisation.
Genetic factors.	Highly signifcant.	Quite signifcant.
Dopamine.	? Overactivity of central dopamine neurons.	? Dopmaine polymorphisms relevant.

Hill (2002) points out that 50 – 80% of "adult offenders have DSM-IV Antisocial Personality Disorder", but the rate of "psychopathy is around 15 – 30%"..

For me in terms of the spectrum of adult offender behaviour, Criminal Autistic Psychopathy and General Psychopathy are at the extreme end, with Antisocial Personality Disorder in the middle and minor offending behaviour at the milder part of the spectrum.

People with either Anti-social Personality Disorder or Criminal Autistic Psychopathy have problems in understanding embarrassment and shame. They both also have problems in understanding "what makes people tick" According to Sacks (1995) they are "unable to appraise a potentially dangerous situation by gauging their own fear, they plough ahead violently, regardless of risk" This occurs in Criminal Autistic Psychopathy and Antisocial Personality Disorder but the deficit is more severe in Criminal Autistic Psychopathy. In my view, there are significant genetic elements in both. They both disregard and violate the rights of others. They both fail to conform to social norms and are deceitful. It was erroneously believed in the past that persons with Autistic Psychopathy could not be deceitful.

While persons with the Autistic Psychopathy subtype in general may have problems with deceit, this certainly is not the case with a number of persons with Criminal Autistic Psychopathy described in this book. They both can disregard the safety of themselves and others. They often show a repeated failure to maintain consistent work behaviour and both show a lack of remorse. They are both very heterogeneous conditions. Clearly a confusion in diagnosis occurs when you have persons with severe Antisocial Personality Disorder who should more accurately be described as having Criminal Autistic Psychopathy. They are both concerned with control and independence for their own behaviour. They both operate on a part object relationship and dehumanise people or just simply use them as objects. They both do not internalise the standard values of society as Dolan and Coid (1993) point out.

Previously in DSM-IV (APA, 1994) patients with these problems were often misdiagnosed as having Antisocial Personality when Criminal Autistic Psychopathy would have been a more appropriate diagnosis. Millon *et al* (2000) point out that "many are shrewd and calculating and struggle to learn the emotional mechanics of interpersonal communication, thus masking their disorder" This of course fits in with the criteria for Criminal Autistic Psychopathy. They also point out that these patients they describe under a Chapter heading of Antisocial Personality "purchase Psychology books explicitly to develop an understanding of human emotional reactions, of "what makes people tick", a "necessary evil" in adapting to an alien world of the empathic and socialised" This is typical of Criminal Autistic Psychopathy and these patients should be classified under this heading and not under the heading of Antisocial Personality. Millon *et al* also points out that "normal subjects react strongly to the emotional dimensions of statements or pictures, but psychopaths do not". This is a problem in General Psychopathy and Criminal Autistic Psychopathy.

"The factor analysis of Hare's (1991) Psychopathy Checklist – Revised produced an impulsive – antisocial factor mirroring the DSM-IV diagnosis of Antisocial Personality Disorder. The analysis yielded a second factor that included items related to emotional and interpersonal relationships (e.g. egocentricity and absence of empathy). This factor is considered by many to represent the core construct of psychopathy, while being relatively neglected by DSM-IV Antisocial Personality Disorder diagnosis" (Widger *et al*, 1996). As Hare and others recognise that many of these patients have major problems with empathy and Criminal Autistic Psychopathy is an empathy disorder. (Hare 1991).

In summary Looney *et al* (2006) point out that "research suggests that a small percentage of antisocial adults exhibit low emotional reactivity (e.g. low autonomic arousal and behavioural reactivity to aversive stimuli), psychopathic traits (i.e. callous unemotional interpersonal style) and a particularly virulent form of antisocial behaviour. These findings have supported a low fearfulness causal model of adult psychopathy (or psychopathic behaviour)". They also point out that "the study of developmental precursors to adult psychopathy has found that childhood conduct problems accompanied by callous unemotional traits are similarly associated with under-reactivity to aversive stimuli and severe conduct problems" They note that "emotional under-reactivity theoretically reduces sensitivity to empathy cues and disrupts the socialisation of conscience and behavioural control" These features would be characteristic of serial killers and persons with Criminal Autistic Psychopathy.

Schizoid Personality, Schizoid Psychopaths, and Criminal Autistic Psychopathy

These persons have been described as loners and were described in 1985 by Patrick Gallwey as Schizoid Psychopaths. I would call many of these as having Criminal Autistic Psychopathy, although there is a considerable overlap between the two categories.

Stone (1998) notes that Thomas Hamilton who killed 16 children plus their teacher in Dunblane Scotland was a "schizoid loner".

Wolff (1998) notes that Schizoid Personality Disorder in childhood lies at one extreme of the autistic spectrum, where it shades into normal personality variation. Wolff (1990) pointed out that Schizoid Personality Disorder in boys showed "solitariness, impaired empathy and emotional detachment, increased sensitivity, rigidity of mental set including the single-minded pursuit of special interests and unusual or odd communication".

All these features are also features of Criminal Autistic Psychopathy. Wolff notes that "adult criminals are likely to include a subgroup with the clinical features of Schizoid Personality. Going back to childhood, whose crimes are likely to be more repetitive, more dangerous, more violent and less comprehensive than those of other offenders" Kozol *et al* (1972) noticed a similar trend. This fits in also with Criminal Autistic Psychopathy.

In Wolff (1990), *Schizoid Disorder,* she noticed an "unusual fantasy life" and antisocial behaviour, which showed "inexplicable and frightening aggression in boys and of fraudulent behaviour and pathological lying in both boys and girls". This is similar to Criminal Autistic Psychopathy. Wolff (1995) in her studies of schizoid girls noted significant antisocial behaviour and that 5 out of 13 had "falsely reported their parents of being cruel to them" and "two had used aliases" It is not true that all persons with Criminal Autistic Psychopathy are incapable of telling lies, although it is true they often have difficulty telling fact from fiction. Wolff (1995) also described a "high rate of criminality in the schizoid women (three times as high as for a comparable group in the general population"). In discussion about Wolff's (1995) book, Gillberg (1996) notes that many of her cases would definitely meet current criteria for Asperger's syndrome (Criminal Autistic Psychopathy). . . [and] that others "would not". I believe Criminal Autistic Psychopathy would be a better name.

Kerr *et al* (2004) noted that aloofness or the absence of friendships predicted later antisocial behaviour. Aloofness and absence of friendships are also central to Criminal Autistic Psychopathy and Schizoid Psychopathy and indeed relationships are also abnormal in General Psychopathy.

The differential diagnosis of Autistic Psychopathy would be Avoidant Personality, Schizoid Personality, and Schizotypal Personality. Persons with Schizoid Personality tend to work as long-distance lorry drivers, night watchmen, or could engage in lone sailing activities.

One major serial killer was a long distance lorry driver. Jung focussed on introversion in relation to these personalities - Jung was an introvert himself with Asperger's syndrome Kretchmer identified a schizoid temperament and noticed that these persons were "brutally frank, or grumpy or vague, or sarcastically ironic, or shy as a mollusc, silent and withdrawn". Criminal Autistic Psychopathy overlaps with Schizoid Personality Disorder, Antisocial Personality Disorder, Paranoid Personality Disorder, Narcissistic Personality Disorder, Schizotypal Personality Disorder, Avoidant Personality Disorder, and Obsessive Compulsive Disorder. According to Stone (1993) in relation to serial killers "one in four are schizoid psychopaths: unempathetic, cold, detached, as well as psychopathic" This would also fit with Criminal Autistic Psychopathy.

Schizoid, schizotypal cases are described by Stone (1993) and in his discussion of Sandra a "phenotypic" Schizotypal patient would now be described as a classic example of a person with Autistic Psychopathy. Stone describes her as eccentric, anxious, with only one friend, "weird", with a high-pitched stilted tone of voice. She was unable to get on people's conversational wavelength. She had major problems with social know-how, empathy, and lacked life skills. Indeed another of Stone's (1993) patients, Paul whom Stone called a "schizoid phenocopy", would also meet the criteria for Autistic Psychopathy. He was a loner, with very poor reciprocal social relations, a night worker who was a great reader, and whose only friends were a "dog and his pet rabbit". He had a "cold aloof affect".

Another of Stone's cases, Shelley whom he described as having "a Schizotypal genophenocopy" also had many Autistic Psychopathy traits, including death anxiety, and being into mysticism, and she was "locked inside her own solipsistic bubble". She showed "autistic logic" and had problems differentiating fact from fiction.

Tantum (1988) has argued that autistic-like abnormalities of social interaction characteristic of Asperger's syndrome (Autistic Psychopathy) "are of a different kind to schizoid abnormalities of social relationship, evinced by emotional detachment introversion and over sensitivity". Tantum (1988) made an interesting point in differentiating Schizoid, Schizotypal and Borderline Personality from Autistic Psychopathy, saying that "their social isolation arose from a failure to make relationships rather than from an abnormality of social interaction". Nevertheless in clinical practice, an overlap between conditions is very much a clinical reality.

What is very interesting is that de River (1956) describes a number of cases as having autistic personality. This was very insightful as this book was written originally in 1949, which was only a few years after Hans Asperger published his work on Autistic Psychopathy. It is interesting that de River ,in describing cases, pointed out that they had "a schizoid type, whole, autistic personality with elements of algolagnia . . . morally frigid and affectively cold" This all fits in nicely with Autistic Psychopathy. The explanations he gives for these activities include Oedipus complex problems etc. These do not explain the phenomena we are dealing with.

For those with Criminal Autistic Psychopathy, their actions are just for pleasure rather than financial gain. There is little doubt that many of these serial killers are sensation seekers or thrill seekers. Boredom drives them then to carry out further killings in order to relieve the boredom and to increase the sensation experience. These killers are often possess sadistic personality traits.

Porter *et al* (2006) point out that "sexual murderers are more likely than other violent offenders to be psychopathic". Because of their empathy deficits, sexual murderers are often largely insensitive to their victims' distress. The victim is regarded as just an object. Sexual murderers lack any shame and disgust. People with Criminal Autistic Psychopathy do not have any feelings of empathy towards their victims particularly when they mutilate the victim. They tend to blame others for their problems.

Prevalence of Schizoid Personality Disorder

Widiger and Rogers (1989) estimated that it was between 0.8% and 1%. This is pretty close to the prevalence of ASDs. Prevalence is not very reliable because there is so much overlap of these disorders.

PARANOID IDEAS, NARCISSISTIC PHENOMENA AND PSYCHOPATHY

Richards (1998) emphasised, correctly, the paranoid-narcissistic problems prevalent in psychopathy. This is also very important in Criminal Autistic Psychopathy. These paranoid/narcissistic problems are common in psychopathic personalities. He emphasises their malicious, predatory, perverse, aggressive features as well as their wish to control and dominate people. Psychopathic behaviour is a pathological form of self-esteem regulation and a way of keeping the fragmented personality together. It is a failed attempt at consolidating one's identity.

Stone's (1993) description of Paranoid Personality contains many traits seen in Criminal Autistic Psychopathy, including suspiciousness, grandiose elements, feeling people are against them, free floating anger and hostility, quarrelousness and a contentious quality. Both can be often mistrustful, humourless and cold emotionally and can be hypersensitive and vengeful. Both misinterpret social cues and can become obsessed with details.

Alexithymia and Autistic Psychopathy

Persons with Alexithymia have problems describing their feelings and emotions and are focussed on concrete external worlds very similar to persons with Criminal Autistic Psychopathy. They also show evidence of somatization disorder, which are physical complaints that cannot be fully explained by known general medical conditions. Persons with Criminal Autistic Psychopathy often show somatization problems both in and out of prison (Fitzgerald, 2004, 2006).

Malignant Alienation and Autistic Psychopathy

This is a concept with many similarities to Autistic Psychopathy introduced by Watts and Morgan (1994). These patients are hard to treat and to like. Watts and Morgan (1994) point out that they are "provocative, unreasonable or over dependent" They are at risk of suicide as indeed are patients with Autistic Psychopathy. The precipitating factors include problems with social relations e.g., rejection. The same occurs with Criminal Autistic Psychopathy. (Fitzgerald, 2005).

Criminal Autistic Psychopathy versus Psychosis

Abell and Hare (2005) showed that "persons with Asperger's syndrome reported higher levels of delusional ideation than the general population . . . mainly of the grandiose or persecutory type". These are quite common in Criminal Autistic Psychopathy. It is easy to see how persons with Criminal Autistic Psychopathy would therefore be easily misdiagnosed as schizophrenia. Age of onset helps, as schizophrenia rarely has an early childhood onset, and Autistic Psychopathy always has an early childhood onset. These delusional beliefs are associated with problems in autobiographical memory in Autistic Psychopathy and problems with self-awareness. Delusional beliefs in schizophrenia appear more severe. Persons with Autistic Psychopathy are "reputed to have fewer delusional beliefs than people experiencing psychosis" (Abel and Hare, 2005). Persons with Autistic Psychopathy have problems separating fact from fiction and this increases the likelihood of delusional experiences. Another factor is that persons with Autistic Psychopathy tend to be negative thinkers. They attempt, through their delusions, to make sense of the puzzling world.

In another study of Asperger's syndrome, Craig et al (2004) showed that persons with Asperger's syndrome had higher scores on a paranoid scale of Fenigstein and Venable (1992) than controls.

Forensic specialists often confuse schizophrenia with Criminal Autistic Psychopathy for the reasons described and this can lead to highly inappropriate treatment.

OVERLAP BETWEEN ATTENTION DEFICIT HYPERACTIVITY, AUTISTIC PSYCHOPATHY AND GENERAL PSYCHOPATHY

When people with Criminal Autistic Psychopathy, Attention Deficit Hyperactivity Disorder, and General Psychopathy are compared to healthy controls, it is clear that they are less socially competent, involve themselves in fewer social activities and have fewer friends. They often show problems in reading social cues. They also show egocentricity and have problems with reciprocal social relationships. I am suggesting there is a considerable overlap between these conditions. While they have been discussed as discrete categories with no overlap, I do believe that from a clinical perspective in the real world there is great overlap.

Lynam (1996, 1998) noted a relationship between Attention Deficit Hyperactivity Disorder and Conduct Disorder and later Psychopathy.

Jensen et al (1997) "showed that children with PDD (Pervasive Developmental Disorder which is an overreaching dimension which includes Autistic Psychopathy) could not be differentiated from children with Attention Deficit Hyperactivity Disorder on scales related to hyperactivity and acting out behaviour. A clinically relevant group of children with PDD and ADHD has been underexposed in the recent literature".

Geurts et al (2004) point out that "the overlap between symptoms of Attention Deficit Hyperactivity Disorder and autism, the large comorbidity, and the finding that a given disorder may be a risk of developing another disorder, are all indications that there is a strong relationship between autism and Attention Deficit Hyperactivity Disorder" Clinicians who diagnose psychopathy commonly miss adult Attention Deficit Hyperactivity Disorder, because they do not assess for it. Multiple diagnosis are more common than not. There is a serious error in DSM-IV (APA, 1994), which does not allow the clinician to diagnose Attention Deficit Hyperactivity Disorder if they first diagnose autism. I believe there is a continuity or spectrum of Attention Deficit Hyperactivity Disorder, Asperger's syndrome/Autistic Psychopathy and non-verbal Learning Disability.

In terms of severity, one can go from Conduct Disorder in children and adolescents to Autistic Personality Disorder/General Psychopathy to Criminal Autistic Psychopathy and finally Psychosis.

Stone (1993) points out that persons with psychopathy overreact to stimuli and show "a superiority, compared with other groups, in the ability to attend to events of particular" interest. This would be typically true of people with Criminal Autistic Psychopathy. There is no doubt that there are psychopathic spectrum disorders or a group of disorders under this umbrella term. Quite a few prisoners with a diagnosis of psychopathy have Criminal Autistic Psychopathy.

SUB CLASSIFICATION OF PSYCHOPATHY

Millon and Davis (1998) identify ten types of psychopath:

(1) unprincipled,
(2) disingenuous,
(3) risk taking,
(4) covetous,
(5) spineless,
(6) explosive,
(7) abrasive,
(8) malevolent,
(9) tyrannical, and
(10) malignant.

Schneider (1958) had a subcategory of psychopathy called explosive, affectionless, and weak willed.

It is not sufficient to use just the word psychopathy, one must also subtype persons with psychopathy. This book adds one more subtype -Criminal Autistic Psychopathy -which would overlap with Millon and Davis' (1998) last three subtypes.

BOUNDARIES OF DIAGNOSTIC CATEGORIES

There is a great deal of fluidity at the borders of many current psychiatric categories, e.g. Autism, Personality Disorder, Psychopathy, Attention Deficit Hyperactivity Disorder, Conduct Disorder, etc. Genes have multiple effects and therefore the same genes could be involved in multiple diagnostic categories. It is certain that in the future, the current boundaries between conditions in DSM-IV (APA, 1994) will be dramatically changed. It is likely that, in future, patients will be placed in five or six different dimensions and not in any single category. Multiple dimensional diagnoses will be the order of the day. Gene profiling will also be critical to diagnosis in the future and to subtyping.

We have achieved now what Aubrey Lewis wished us to achieve back in 1953. He wrote that "until the category (of psychopathic personality) is . . shown to be characterised by specified abnormality of psychological functions, it will not be possible to consider those who fall within it to be unhealthy". We have achieved this now.

GENETICS AND PSYCHOPATHY

Autistic Psychopathy is a highly heritable disorder with heritability estimates of over 90%. It is not surprising that Viding (2004) notes that: "the personality traits at the core of psychopathy are more highly heritable than other personality traits". Criminal Autistic Psychopathy subtype is also highly heritable. There is a need for future research in studies of gene environment interaction.

Hyman(2002) stated that "almost all behaviour is conditioned partly by the interaction of many, many genes, plus environment, plus something we generally do not like to think about but that is very important – chance. Given that the wiring up of some hundred trillion synapses can't happen identically even in identical twins, the prediction of even the most genetic of mental illnesses, such as autism, can only be probabilistic".

Blair *et al* (2006) state that in children, examining almost 3,500 twin pairs within the Twins Early Development Study (TEDS), the callous and unemotional component of psychopathic tendencies was indexed at age 7 (Viding, Blair, Moffitt, and Plomin, 2005). This study revealed a significant group heritability of $h^2 g = .67$ and no shared environmental influence on the callous-unemotional component; i.e. genetic factors account for two-thirds of the difference between the callous-unemotional probands and the population.

What I believe is inherited is the empathy deficits of Autistic Psychopathy and, or the novelty seeking, sensation seeking associations of Attention Deficit Hyperactivity Disorder.

It is likely that multiple genes of small effect are involved with in addition gene: gene interactions. For Blair *et al* (2006) the causes of psychopathy are "genes, physical/sexual abuse and brain damage (for example, from alcohol/drug abuse during pregnancy or birth complications)". I agree with this.

CRITICISM OF PSYCHOPATHY

Gunn (1998) states that "in all my work, I do not use the noun "psychopath", the adjective "psychopathic" or the phrase "psychopathic disorder". In my opinion these terms confuse and mislead". Gunn (1998) states that "the term psychopath can soon be consigned to history books, novels, films, and the vernacular". Indeed the opposite has happened as set out in this book for good scientific reasons.

Miller (1991) criticises the psychopathy concept as "hurtful and defeating . . . diagnoses which ensure neglect, mishandling, and brutality" Any diagnosis can be misused but psychopathy does describe real human beings who show dehumanised behaviour and we ignore it at our peril. If a person misunderstands a concept, that is their responsibility. Not using a concept does not mean it will go away and that it will cease to exist. Misunderstanding needs education not deletion. Blackburn (1988) describes psychopaths as being a "mythical entity" Those suffering at the hands of Jeffrey Dahlmer a serial killer with Criminal Autistic Psychopathy, would be slow to state (if they were alive) that psychopathy was too harsh a diagnosis.

Mawson (1983) describes the problems with the concept of psychopathic disorder. He points out that "psychiatrists disagree about the term and its diagnosis in particular cases. Secondly, the term was described as logically defective, inferring mental disorder from antisocial behaviour, while explaining the latter by the former. A third criticism of the concept was that moral explanations of the behaviour were being ousted by medico-scientific ones"

Mawson further notes "another criticism of the term was that it approved stigmatic, harmful and indelible, and that it made those so labelled more difficult to handle". He also pointed out that the "Mental Health Act 1983 (in the UK) defined psychopathic disorder as a persistent disorder or disability of mind (whether or not including significant impairment of intelligence) which results in abnormally aggressive or seriously irresponsible conduct"

Viding (2004) points out that the "personality aspect of psychopathy is stable across the life span". Therefore, why delete it? Criminal Autistic Psychopathy also occurs across the lifespan.

Stone (1998) points out that Sadistic Personality Disorder was criticised by people for "medicalization of evil deeds". Many of the criticisms of the concept of psychopathy are really due to "political correctness" and the denial of evil, which is largely genetically inherited in most of these cases. I do not agree with this political correctness attitude, as it gets rid of a valid and reliable diagnostic category.

Indeed not all social commentators are happy with these discussions about children. Sereny (2005) stated that "to assume that a three year old child shows symptoms of criminality seems to me so ridiculous that I can hardly find words for it. I am shocked by the mere idea".

My view is that General Psychopathy and Criminal Autistic Psychopathy are useful concepts. We can identify them in Forensic Psychiatry. They increase our understanding of persons who have committed crimes and are of predictive importance. They tend to be linked with recidivism.

LANGUAGE AND PSYCHOPATHY

There are problems with language in persons with General Psychopathy. They often show a disassociation between their spoken language, emotional processing and non-verbal behaviour. This has been long recognised. Hiatt and Newman (2006) note that in examining the history of psychopathy Ronald Blackburn noted that "by analogy with semantic aphasia (it was) hypothesised that the psychopaths defect was deep, probably biologically based disorder disturbing the integration of experience and resulting in a pathological loss of meaning".

Primary psychopaths - a phrase used by Clekley (1950) have what he described as "semantic aphasia". According to Millon *et al* (2000), this means a "class of disorders related to the understanding or production of language". This seems very close to persons with Criminal Autistic Psychopathy who have pragmatic language problems.

Blair (2006) in *Handbook of Psychopathy* points out that "individuals with psychopathy have been found to be more impaired in some forms of semantic processing. These effects have been related, through recent fMRI work, to reduced activity in right anterior temporal gyrus and surrounding cortex in individuals with psychopathy. Of course given the unclear relevance of these semantic difficulties to abstract word processing to the emergence of the disorder, it is possible that they reflect educational differences between the individuals with psychopathy and comparison individuals". I believe this is genetic and not, by in large, environmental.

Primary psychopathy is very close to Criminal Autistic Psychopathy. Millon *et al* (1998) pointed out that "Clekley believed . . that psychopaths suffer an inborn inability to understand and express the meaning of emotional experience". This is equivalent to Criminal Autistic Psychopathy. They have problems understanding the emotional meaning of experience.

According to Hiatt and Newman (2006), Hare (1986) pointed out that "Clekley long held that the speech of psychopaths appears to be a mechanically correct artefact that masks a semantic disorder in which the formal, semantic, and affective components of language are dissociated from one another" General psychopaths have problems with processing the emotional aspects of language and indeed Herve, Hayes, and Hare (2003) pointed out that "incarcerated psychopaths do not understand or make effective use of the emotional content of language" Indeed emotional feelings can be absent from their language. This also occurs in Criminal Autistic Psychopathy.

Hare and Jutai (1988) in relation to psychopathy stated that "weak or unusual lateralisation of language function, and that psychopathy may have fewer left hemisphere resources for processing language than do normal individuals". Hiatt *et al* (2006) point out that persons with "psychopathy show poor use of secondary or contextual aspects of language" as so persons with Criminal Autistic Psychopathy.

Problems with abstract reasoning are common. The relevance of "weak or unusual lateralisation of language function" is not clear but there is some evidence that "manual skills may show an atypical (less lateralisation) pattern in autism (Smith, 2000). Further studies in this area are needed. Persons with Criminal Autistic Psychopathy are often clumsy and have an awkward walk.

In General Psychopathy, the atypical cerebral asymmetry of the brain would appear to be quite important in understanding the language problems. They use unusual cerebral language processing which may underpin their unusual emotional relationships. Atypical brain processing and atypical language and emotional processing maybe a feature of General Psychopathy. There is less language processed in the left hemisphere in general psychopaths, than in persons without psychopathy. This is further evidence of atypical cerebral asymmetry including problems with communication between cerebral hemispheres.

Oberman (*Science Daily*, 205/04) points out that the mirror neuron system is involved in higher cognitive processes like language. It is likely that the mirror neuron system is malfunctioning in General Psychopathy and Criminal Autistic Psychopathy (http//www.sciencedaily.com.205/04).

Baumeister (1997) notes that in general psychotherapy that perpetrators use "linguistic tendencies, again, at the expense of downplaying the victims suffering".

There is some evidence for this and Blair, Mitchell (2005) note the "reduced affective input to linguistic processing". This is part of the autistic narrative style.

France (1998) points out that criminals have "a husky, creaky, rough sound aided by considerable muscular tension of the neck and shoulders, and use inappropriate vocal volume either too loud or too soft, usually the latter" Unusual tones of voice are common in Criminal Autistic Psychopathy.

Persons with Criminal Autistic Psychopathy tend to have poorer capacity to communicate through language, and a poorer capacity of sharing emotional feelings and for comforting. They are also poorer at understanding non-verbal behaviour.

In General Psychopathy and Criminal Autistic Psychopathy, there is an overlap in Speech and Language problems.

Chapter 4

ASPERGER'S SYNDROME/CRIMINAL AUTISTIC PSYCHOPATHY AND VIOLENCE

Right from the beginning of the discussion on Autistic Psychopathy, the link with aggression and violence was made.

Uta Frith (1991) in her translation of Hans Asperger's 1944 paper states that Fritz V, one of Hans Asperger's patients was "aggressive" and "lashed out with anything he could get hold of (once a hammer)" and he "attacked other children" and "appeared to "enjoy people being angry". The next patient Harro L. was an "inveterate liar" in that: "he told "long fantastic stories". This challenges the notion that persons with Asperger's Syndrome cannot lie, but some can and this was recognised from the very fist discussions of Autistic Psychopathy (Asperger's syndrome).

Hans Asperger also mentioned "autistic acts of malice". Frith (1991) writes that: "these acts appear to be calculated" and could be "sadistic acts" and "delight in malice". Asperger also wrote that: "sadistic traits" are frequent. One boy with Autistic Psychopathy said:

> "Mummy, I shall take a knife one day and push it into your heart, then blood will spurt out and this will cause a great stir" and "it would be nice to be a wolf. Then I could rip apart sheep and people, and then blood will flow".

This has many echoes of the adults I describe in this book and has echoes of Criminal Autistic Psychopathy experimentation.

Hans Asperger also noticed the perversions these people often show. One can see how right Asperger was when one reads about the murderers in this book. Those with Criminal Autistic Psychopathy perversions are associated with empathy deficits.

I do not agree with Uta Frith (1991) that: "autistic people are not interested in hurting". They can premeditate and form intentions and indeed juries in the Western World have taken this view. Frith (1991) points out that they don't have "an active theory of mind". There are all degrees of capacity to have an understanding or theory of other people's minds as is well illustrated in the cases descried in this book. Indeed there is no doubt some of them have a theory of mind.

Frith describes their behaviour as "innocent detached curiosity". Nothing could be further from the truth in the cases described in my book. She also emphasised the "lack of common sense" as a defence but this would not get any of the cases described in this book "off the hook". In my experience (Fitzgerald, 2004) most persons with Autistic Psychopathy are highly moral and the most law abiding people on the face of the earth. Nevertheless there is a subcategory of Asperger's Syndrome – Persons with Criminal Autistic Psychopathy who are extremely dangerous and can be serial killers. Frith (1991) states that: "typically the Asperger individual, when apprehended does not seem to feel guilt, does not try to conceal or excuse. What he or she did and may actually describe details with shocking openness". This is what this book sets out to show in persons with Criminal Autistic Psychopathy, e.g. Peter Kurten, Albert de Salvo, etc. Again it's not all or nothing as serial killers in their earlier days do make more efforts to escape detection.

Shea and Mesibov (2005), in referring to Howlin's (1997, 2000) work, state that persons with Asperger's Syndrome who have 'run-ins' with the law do not have "malicious or unscrupulous motives". In the subgroup of Asperger's Syndrome Criminal Autistic Psychopathy subtypes studied in this book nothing could be further from the truth in real life situations. I wonder how the victim's families would respond being told that the murderer or indeed a serial killer was not "malicious or unscrupulous". Shea *et al* (2005) who put Asperger "crimes" in inverted commas – I assume to suggest they are not real crimes but various special interests. Limited understanding of appropriate sexual social behaviour plays a role in criminal Autistic Psychopathy. In the *Handbook of Autism and Pervasive Developmental Disorders* criminality is regarded as such a minor topic that it is only given one page in a handbook of over 1300 pages. This is extraordinary particularly on a topic of massive importance to the public.

Allen *et al* (2006) studied offending by persons with Asperger's Syndrome in a population of 1.2 million. They identified 126 people of whom 33 were identified as having offended. The mean age committing the first offence was 25.8 years. These persons showed a history of verbal aggression (75%) and inappropriate sexual behaviour (69%). In terms of offending 81% showed violent conduct and 19% sexual offences. The offences included arson, murder, stalking, and violent assault. They showed that predisposing factors included overriding obsessions (44%) and social naivety (88%).

For Allen *et al* (2006), precipitating factors included social rejection (69%) and sexual rejection (50%). This finding fits very well with the more serious offending with Criminal Autistic Psychopathy, which I will describe later.

ASPERGER'S SYNDROME – CRIMINAL AUTISTIC PSYCHOPATHY SUBGROUP

O'Brien and Bell (2004), note that Asperger described in his cases "odd and bizarre antisocial behaviours". Lorna Wing in Asperger's Syndrome (1991) noted, "a small minority have a history of rather bizarre antisocial acts, perhaps because of their lack of empathy" Asperger himself according to them described "a number of violent, aggressive and antisocial acts carried out by his subjects. A child who was obsessed by poisons stole substantial quantities of cyanide from a locked school store; happily, this was discovered before he had an opportunity to try it out" This latter interest in chemicals combined with an apparent lack of empathy appears to be not uncommon and a cause for some concern. In this book Graham

Young did carry out his poisoning plans. One of Lorna Wing's original groups injured a boy in the course of his chemistry experiments.

Mawson and colleagues' (1985) subject also had interest in poisons and "admitted to contemplating poisoning a peer after an altercation". They point out that: "in Tantum's 1988 sample of 60 socially isolated individuals about 50% had committed a criminal act and only 22% were charged". They also point out that in persons with autism "offences did not tend to be instrumental in that there was no direct gain to the individual nor did it appear to be a means to an end. Secondly the persons with autism were significantly less likely to use drugs or alcohol and substance misuse. Thirdly persons with autism had committed offences during daylight hours while other subjects had offended by day and night. They also note that some persons with autism are naïve and this accounts for their activities, others don't like to be changed from their routines, other misinterpret the social interactional behaviour" of others.

Tantum (1991) discusses the "callous individuals" among his Asperger group of persons. This is a very appropriate description and in line with clinical reality. He also mentioned "unpredictable violence". Tantum (1991) mentions four people who were fire setters and had Asperger's syndrome. He also stated that: "sexual excitement – is rarely shown by people with Asperger's syndrome. Sexual offending is usually rare". I don't believe this is always so and believe I have demonstrated this in this book. Kohn *et al* (1998) estimated the prevalence of aggression in Asperger's Syndrome to be around 20%. Siponmaa *et al* (2001) in a study of 135 young offenders estimated that 30% had a possible diagnosis of PDD (Pervasive Developmental Disorder which includes autism and Asperger's syndrome) including 4% with definite Asperger's syndrome. Barry-Walsh and Mullen (2004) in discussing Murrie *et al* (2002) discussed the issue of reduced empathy and the insanity defence. They speculated that: "insanity and competence a key issue might prove to be the extent to which suggested reality of those with Asperger's Syndrome differed from other individuals". Clearly persons with Asperger's Syndrome do have problems in separating fact from fiction and have a different reality. They know "the nature and quality of their acts and know that they are wrong" Then they are not within the McNaghten rules of excuse for their crimes. These rules relate to mental responsibility for acts. Barry-Walsh *et al* (2004) describe an 'Asperger' arsonist with a fascination for looking at flickering flames. The next person they describe with Asperger's Syndrome was a stalker and another was charged with assault on his father, while another person with Asperger's Syndrome was charged with sexual offences because of an inappropriate approach to a woman. He did not understand that what he was doing was wrong. Barry-Walsh *et al* (2004) conclude that: "the core features of Asperger's Syndrome and how they determine what the individual knows and understands of the world should form a basis for sophisticated assessment of the issues of disability and legal insanity".

Scragg and Shah (1994) showed a very considerably increased rate of Asperger's Syndrome at 2% in Broadmoor Special Hospital. I have no doubt that they are absolutely right. *Prevalence of Asperger's Syndrome in a Secure Hospital* was a landmark publication showing the relationship between those incarcerated for crime and Asperger's Syndrome or what I call Criminal Autistic Psychopathy.

Volkmar and Klin (2000) note that: "in their review of the literature Ghaziuddin, Tsai, and Ghaziuddin (1991) found no support" for an association of Asperger's Syndrome and violence. I am showing in this book that one should be very wary of accepting this reassurance. Just because the rate of criminal violence by persons with Asperger's Syndrome is lower than the general population rate does not make it less serious and of course there is a lot of violence in Asperger's Syndrome that does not come to the attention of the legal system.

Clinically we see a great deal of aggression in families with an Asperger member. When you look at the total population of 12 to 15 year olds, 16 to 19 year olds, and 20 to 24 year olds, Ghaziuddin quotes figures of "about 6, 6.5, and 7%" being involved in rape, robbery, and assault. Clearly lower rates are found for populations with Asperger's syndrome. This does not mean that the violence in Asperger's Syndrome is therefore not a problem. In these small subgroups of patients with Asperger's Syndrome/Criminal Autistic Psychopathy the violence is of extraordinary severity and includes serial killers.

Tantum (2000) emphasises the unusual stimuli that can set off aggression in persons with Asperger's Syndrome including thinking about past insults, "displaced" on to someone else and "uninhibited by empathic response to the intended victims fear". Persons with Asperger's Syndrome (Criminal Autistic Psychopathy subtype) who commit crimes want total control and dominance over another human being. They tend to fail in the routine interpersonal relationships and are rejected because of their poor capacity for reciprocal social relationships. This can lead to hundreds of deep hurts because of these rejections and lead to thoughts of vengeance on people. Unfortunately they can then take out their vengeance on random people.

Klin and Volkmar (2000) in discussing the association between "violence and criminal behaviour" and Asperger's Syndrome state that the data "do not support such associations" I believe that I have shown precisely the opposite conclusions in the persons described in this book. It would be very dangerous and lead to further death by killing by denying the association between Autistic Psychopathy and very serious crime. It would mean that Forensic Psychiatry would not look out for this diagnosis and the current situation would continue.

Siponmaa *et al* (2001), in a study of juvenile and young adult mentally disordered offenders, found a rate of Autism Spectrum Disorder of 27% using DSM-IV criteria and 10% with Asperger's Syndrome using Gillberg's (1991) criteria.

Siponmaa *et al* state that: "in the United Kingdom, Scragg and Shah have reported that the rate of Asperger's Syndrome in patients in adult forensic security hospitals (1.5% - 2.3%) is higher than in the general population (0.4%)" In their study of 130 young patients aged 15 to 22 years they found that: "15% of the whole group had a definite PDD diagnosis, and 12% had a probable PDD diagnosis. The occurrence of PDDNOS was particularly high. Autistic disorder was not found in any case". "Sixteen individuals had committed arson. The diagnosis of PDDNOS and Asperger's Syndrome were statistically more frequent in the arson group than it was in the other crime groupings. This was the only significant relationship between type of crime and diagnosis that was found". They also point out that: "the definite case of Asperger's Syndrome 3% was higher than that in the general population 0.4%, but was of the same order of magnitude as that found by Scragg and Shah (1.5% - 2.3%) who studied adult subjects in a secure hospital who were undergoing forensic psychiatric treatment".

In Hare, Gould, Mills, and Wing (1999) study of maximum-security hospitals, the rate of Autism Spectrum Disorder was 2.4%. There is clear evidence of an association between Asperger's Syndrome / Autistic Psychopathy and criminal behaviour but it's more in the subcategory of Asperger's Syndrome called Criminal Autistic Psychopathy.

Critically Harbort *et al*, showed that: "dysfunctional development in primary socialisation processes could be observed for 89.1% of the sample killers". This is what you would expect in Criminal Autistic Psychopathy. They also showed greater "signs of alienation, social maladjustment" than single murderers. Sex was often very important. They were "more socially isolated or alienated individuals. They have higher rates of unemployment and previous convictions" This would make them more likely to be Criminal Autistic Psychopathy as well as other forms of psychopathy.

Hansen (1998) correctly draws attention to Ole Sylvester Jorgensen's book *Mellem Autisme Og Normalitet (Between autism and Normality)*, and points out that it is precisely this zone that many psychopathic criminals find themselves" (Hansen, 1998).

Murrie et al (2002) again describe a "small subset of Asperger's Syndrome patients (who) come into contact with the legal system due to their social impairments and idiosyncratic interests". They noted their "cold, heartless and remorseless behaviour", "egocentricity and shallow affect", "naiveties", "immediate confession" and "deficient shame" They make the very critical point of the difficulty of distinguishing psychotic delusion and perception from perception and belief in persons with Asperger's syndrome, which may be due to interpersonal empathy deficits. Clearly the psychiatric history is different in Asperger's Syndrome from schizophrenia and is not associated with the mental deterioration that you see in schizophrenia. Delusions in persons with Asperger's Syndrome are less severe than in persons with schizophrenia.

Abell and Hare (2005) point out that persons with Asperger's Syndrome have "relatively high levels of delusional ideation, primarily grandiose or persecutory" but "less than people with psychosis".

The cases that Murrie describes included one of arson, three cases of sexual offences, and one of attempted murder. Baron-Cohen (1988) described a young man with Asperger's Syndrome who assaulted a 71 year old woman.

Everall and Le Couter (1990) described fire setting in an adolescent with Asperger's syndrome. Persons with Asperger's Syndrome who offend usually don't have the long list of offences committed in comparison to persons with non-Asperger's Syndrome delinquent histories. The crimes are atypical and they may have only one or two contacts with the law in their life. Of course the one legal contact can throw up a large number of serial killings. Christopher Gillberg (2002), the foremost clinician and researcher in the area of Asperger's Syndrome stated that: "he knew a few people with Asperger's Syndrome . . . who actually persecuted people".

Howlin (1997) stated that there "is little of any significant association between autism and criminal offending" This statement makes no sense when you examine the literature on this topic as already done. Howlin (1997) describes a boy who put the gas in the house at full blast as an experiment. Nevertheless she notes that: "a 13 year old boy diagnosed with Asperger's Syndrome murdered a 85 year old woman on the way to church without any motivation". She also notes that Mawson (1985) "reports on a 44 year old man with Asperger's Syndrome who committed to Broadmoor Special Hospital after attacking a baby. This followed a series of other attacks including stabbing. The attacks seemed to be related to the obsession with getting a girlfriend, his dislike of certain styles of dress, and his dislike of the noise of crying. He also had a fascination with poisons".

Howlin (1997) concludes that: "there is no reason to suppose that people with autism are more prone to committing offences than anyone else". I wonder what Jeffrey Dahlmer's victims would say to this view. These are the more organised type of murderers As I have shown in this book persons with Criminal Autistic Psychopathy often show a great deal of planning in their acts.

PERSONS WITH ASPERGER'S SYNDROME AS VICTIMS

There is a general agreement that persons with Asperger's Syndrome are far more likely to be victims than to be perpetrators. The serious perpetrators are better defined as Criminal Autistic Psychopathy. The majority of persons with Asperger's Syndrome that I have been involved with clinically have been bullied to a greater or lesser extent in schools and indeed in later life. The bullying has been of the most vicious, relentless and unbelievable kind. Persons who are likely to engage in bullying are on the look out for potential victims. The person with Asperger's Syndrome is the perfect victim in the schoolyard particularly. They are noticed to be slightly different, have poor relationship skills, to be standing alone or apart from other groups, or to engage in monotonous discussions about topics of their own interest, which bore other boys or girls in the playground. They have problems with empathy, problems with social skills, problems reading non-verbal behaviour or body language, problems in understanding how other peers minds are working all lead to major problems in reciprocal social relationships and to major interpersonal difficulties which end up with the person with Asperger's Syndrome being rejected, being called names, and being bullied.

I have also observed adolescents with Asperger's Syndrome getting into trouble with the law because a streetwise peer suggested to them that they should steal something from a shop and they go along and do it. Persons with Asperger's Syndrome have very considerable difficulties with social distance and have major difficulties in making relationships with girls that they hope with lead to a boyfriend / girlfriend situation. They have problems with the language to engage in these courting rituals. They may inappropriately touch a girl and be reported to the police because of this. They have difficulty understanding the non-verbal cues of the girl that they are approaching. It is not that they wanted to do something wrong but that they didn't understand the social know-how of how to do it right (Harpur *et al*, 2004; 2006).

Denis Debbaudt from the Debbaudt Detective Agency has many good tips on how to manage these situations. Debbaudt (2002) suggests the basic information that one may wish to give to one's neighbours to avoid a child or adolescent with Asperger's Syndrome being misunderstood by them. He also discusses how school based awareness of Asperger's Syndrome can be increased and why all members of staff need to be educated about these matters. Persons with Asperger's Syndrome need to be taught the appropriate way to interact with the police should they come into contact with them. He also emphasises the importance of having an "Autism Emergency Contact Handout Model" which includes Name, Date of Birth, Photograph, Contact Numbers, Special Characteristics, Places the person likes, and Patient's special interest, likes, dislikes – approach and de-escalation techniques.

Clearly Police Colleges need also to educate future policemen about Asperger's Syndrome and how it presents. Debbaudt emphasised the importance of having a secure home to prevent wandering. Debbaudt also has tips for law enforcement officers mainly focussing on persons with autism, general reactions etc. He suggested talking to them with brief sentences that are clear and concrete. He suggested not to use metaphorical language. He tells them of their sensitivity to touch and their hypersensitivity to encroachment or being put in with significant groups of other prisoners. He also tells them not to expect rapid responses to questions.

Chapter 5

CRIMINAL AUTISTIC PSYCHOPATHY AND GENERAL PSYCHOPATHY AS A DISORDER OF SELF

DEFINITION OF SELF

"The self as we know is a harmonious blend of internal and external representations, central organising principles, emotions, determinations of need, value, and risk, application of appropriate automatic movements, and visions of the past and future. The success of this integrated self in answering the questions of daily life and the consistency with which self representations organise adaptive behaviour will determine, in great part, what we find when we turn our gaze inwards." (Viamontes *et al*, 2004)

The self-awareness problems of autism were discussed by Kanner (1973).

Autistic Psychopathy is a disorder of the self and persons with Autistic Psychopathy have a severely damaged sense of self, as well as other awareness. Beitman and Nair (2004) point out that:

"Like all psychological functions, the human ability to step back, observe oneself, and to understand the inner workings of another mind, requires some formatting within the brain."

In a way the capacity for self-observation is one of the greatest human achievements. When the self is disordered this capacity to self observe is reduced. This is critical in persons with Criminal Autistic Psychopathy who are serial killers.

Persons with Criminal Autistic Psychopathy have problems differentiating self from other and fact from fiction. Children with Autistic Psychopathy have problems with mirror self-recognition. They develop this rather slowly compared to the average child. Non-autistic children have pretend games, which improve their social skills. Pretend games are delayed in children with Autistic Psychopathy. Persons with Autistic Psychopathy have problems with a sense of time and are often very focussed exclusively on the present. Dahlmer the serial killer was a concrete thinker, had to act out, could not do think symbolically.

The language problems including semantic pragmatic problems interfere with the development of an authentic sense of self. This then also interferes with reality testing and capacity for self-awareness. Without proper language development thinking is restricted, limited, concrete and narrow. This is the case in Criminal Autistic Psychopathy.

The person with Autistic Psychopathy has a fragmented unintegrated emotional life. This is at the heart of the serial killer with Criminal Autistic Psychopathy. The serial killer who has Criminal Autistic Psychopathy does not have a capacity for integrating emotions and forming a clear sense of self. In a way they are all over the place from an emotional point of view and this is due to the problems with normal neural connections in the brain. The neurons in the brain are not properly connected. This can make them into robotic serial killers.

It is possible that some serial killers have developed abnormal neural connections because of gross neglect in the first two years of life. The other alternative explanation is that they may have genetic factors operating but also gross neglect – a case of nature and nurture.

Children experiencing gross neglect in their first few years for example in Eastern European orphanages appear to have serious neural connectivity deficit not totally dissimilar to those with the largely genetic Autistic Psychopathy. They have gross damage to their sense of self, to their capacity for information processing, and serious damage to the brain including the prefrontal cortex. They have very poor capacity for emotional processing.

Persons with General Psychopathy and Criminal Autistic Psychopathy have problems with reflective mentalisation.

Beitman, Nair and Viamontes (2004) point out that reflective self-functioning refers to "the automatic processes by which people take note of their internal experiences and the possibilities going on in the mind of another person, and come to a conclusion about how to respond." Reflective self-functioning is poor in persons with Criminal Autistic Psychopathy.

Persons with Autistic Psychopathy tend to live in the present and have a poor sense of passing of time or of the past or future. They often have a very good memory for facts. This reflects Dahlmer a serial killer and many serial killers. Serial killers commonly blame others for their problems as do persons with Autistic Psychopathy.

Stuss (2004) states that:

> "stripped of our ability to mentalise, we are at the mercy of what is currently being experienced and perceived in the external world."

This may very well relate to the situation with Criminal Autistic Psychopathy.

The brain of the autistic person in some ways and particularly in relation to serial killers has not evolved as far as people without Autistic Psychopathy.

> "The serial killers appear to have problems with autobiographical memory with the navigation of the self through time as well as dealing with the past particularly in an emotional sense and problems looking at the future". (Viamontes *et al*, 2004)

In terms of evolutionary change it is at a much earlier stage of development particularly in relation to social and emotional issues.

These deficits in autobiographical memory, interfere with the capacity to develop an authentic sense of self. They lack the capacity for social learning or learning from experience. they are driven by internal perverse sadistic desires and give very little attention to their environments. They have a fragmented perverse self.

The sense of self is located in the prefrontal cortex:

"It facilitates multidimensional associations, and provides the means to navigate through time. While many parts of the brain function to define the now, the prefrontal cortex tempers the present moment with an autobiographical, analytic synthesis of the past, as well as projection of the self into the future". (Viamontes et al, 2004)

Therefore abnormalities of the prefrontal cortex are critical in serial killers. Persons such as serial killers don't have the ability to fit into the social order and to inhibit murderous impulses and have reduced capacity for free will and reduced capacity for choice in their daily actions and are driven by their murder lust.

They have very little capacity to stop killing. They lack normal social principals and lack an understanding of the future. They are at an earlier stage of evolutionary development with their automatic killing responses. This is Criminal Autistic Psychopathy. They are very much "here and now" people.

The Criminal Autistic Psychopath has difficulty with reflective thinking. They have a diminished sense of self, a fragmented self, which is unable to put a break on their impulses.

Because of a malfunctioning cortex in Criminal Autistic Psychopathy, there is very poor emotional information processing, poor ability to inhibit impulse, very concrete thinking with poor capacity for mentalisation and simplistic narrow thinking style.

This is typical of the killer with Criminal Autistic Psychopathy. Therefore internally they only have one option and that is to kill. They are unable to learn from experience and are locked into rigid inappropriate patterns of behaviour. In a way they are like automatons in terms of serial killing. Once they get into this mode of behaviour then they are locked into it. In serial killers the frontal lobe is malfunctioning and therefore reduces their choices of action indeed gets rid of choice altogether and leaves them with only one option and that is to kill. For practical purposes there is greatly reduced free will even though that they don't have schizophrenia. The serial killer with Criminal Autistic Psychopathy in a way has a fairly simple social environment that is to find a person to kill and then to kill them. They don't take the complexity of the social situation into account or the feelings of the victim.

Dopamine is critical for reward and for the focussing on matter of great importance to an individual i.e. a victim to be killed. If there is too much Dopamine this focus can be overwhelming, i.e. in finding a victim to kill. Viamontes et al (2004) also point out in Chapter Two of their book that "the appetitive self, powered by the expectation of reward, emerges triumphant and suppresses other self representations. There is no consideration of consequences, internalised rules, or intimations of the future when the appetitive self is in the ascendancy" This is the situation in which the serial killer is in. The appetitive self is linked to the reward system of the brain.

Further self-other confusion is caused by persons with Autistic Psychopathy tending to psychologically merge with other people. There is poor self – other differentiation. At times they see others as part of themselves. This merger is facilitated by making the other person unconscious through drugs and under their control as in the case of the serial killer Dahlmer.

Zimmer (2005) in reference to Sarah Jane Blakemore's work discusses the anterior insula "located on the brain surface not far from the ear. It is possible that the anterior insula helps to designate some information as relating to ourselves instead of to other people". This area of the brain may be also malfunctioning in serial killers because at times they do have difficulty separating themselves from others and indeed tend to fuse with people. The medial prefrontal cortex according to Zimmer "may draw together perceptions and memories of self and combine them into an ongoing feeling of being oneself". In the Carl Zimmer article in *Scientific American* Heatherton states that "he suspects that the area [medial prefrontal cortex] may bind together all the perceptions and memories that help to produce a sense of self, creating a unitary feeling of who we are" The serial killer has a deficient sense of self and a deficient sense of the other. "God" or the capacity to judge good and evil is in the frontal lobe.

Hobson and Meyer J. A. (2005) point out that children with autism have "relative lack of self-consciousness, sometimes obliviousness towards others, and difficulties with aspects of social understanding such as those expressed in pragmatic language and the use of 'I' and 'you'" They also have abnormalities in their "engagement with others attitudes and actions towards a shared world, their use of personal pronouns, and their understanding of mental states in themselves and others" They are impaired from a biological point of view in the specifically "human form of social connectedness: the propensity to identify with another person, that is, to relate to the actions and attitudes of someone else from the other's perspective or stance in such a way that the child assumes or assimilates the others orientation towards the world, including towards the self". They point out that "the mechanism of identification is weak" in autism and indeed criminal autistic psychopathy.

Gerard Bosch (1970) notes that in autism there is "a delay in the constituting of the other person as someone in whose place I can put myself … and in the constituting of a common sphere of existence, in which things do not simply refer to me but also to others." This is central to Criminal Autistic Psychopathy.

In terms of sense of self and identity the pronominal reversal characteristic of Autistic Psychopathy has been recognised from the beginning and is a feature of the confusion of self and other. They have greatly diminished understanding of themselves and others and this is one of the reasons they are sometimes misdiagnosed as borderline personality disorder. The language problems are central to this deficit in autism. They tend to get stuck in superficial meaning, of superficial understanding of themselves, others and social situations. They have huge difficulties in seeing subtexts of conversations, which are often the most important aspects of communication. They are operating in a rather primitive concrete poorly symbolised world. This was probably a world in which our primitive ancestors lived in. It was a world before the vast development of the neo-cortex. It was probably a very visual world. It was probably a world in which primitive language was beginning to develop.

Morrison (2004) points out that Richard Macek, a serial killer, had "a peculiar combination of male and female characteristics" Identity diffusion and androgyny is a central feature of persons with Criminal Autistic Psychopathy who are egocentric, narcissistic, and grandiose. They have a poor sense of self and other and operate on a part-object relationship that is where others are dehumanised and simply there to be an abuser and killer.

Chapter 6

PSYCHOLOGICAL ASPECTS OF (AUTISTIC) PSYCHOPATHY

VIOLENCE INHIBITION MECHANISM

Blair (1995) emphasised the Violence Inhibition Mechanism and stated that that this was impaired in psychopathy. Violence Inhibition Mechanism is a mechanism for controlling aggression in humans, dogs, etc. The individual submits and the aggressor withdraws. In normal life an aggressor sees that another person is upset and disturbed and stops their aggressive behaviour. This does not happen in psychopathy. Persons with psychopathy have reduced sensitivity to distressing upsetting cues from others. Blair and Frith (2000) claim that this is due to a malfunctioning of the amygdala. This fits also with Criminal Autistic Psychopathy.

According to Nigg (2006), in discussing temperament, he stated that the research evidence indicates:

(a) "A problem in a functional violence inhibition system designed to evoke empathy and detection of sadness / fear (submission) in others, and
(b) rooted in the amygdala."

Nigg suggests, in relation to psychopathic tendencies, that there is a:

"temperamentally low withdrawal response, especially low fear and low affiliation. This pathway is hypothesized to include low physiological arousal both at baseline and low electrodermal responses to possible punishment. When low fear is apparent early in life, it may disrupt the formation of guilt, conscience or concern about punishment".

This occurs in Criminal Autistic Psychopathy and General Psychopathy.

Viding (2004) noted that children of age 3.5 years make judgements "between moral (victim-based) and conventional (social-disorder based) transgressions" Persons with psychopathy tend not to think about the victim when deciding to do something or not to do it. Persons with psychopathy have problems in recognising "fearful and sad vocal affects" (Blair *et al* 2002). Persons with psychopathy are relatively insensitive to punishments. They have great difficulty learning from experience. If they do something violent and are punished the punishment has no effect. Indeed they are more likely to feel victims than perpetrators. They are therefore insensitive to social norms. They also ignore positive responses but to a lesser degree.

Blair *et al* (2005) noted that individuals with psychopathy had problems recognising sad and fearful facial expressions and showed "reduced autonomic activity to sad facial expression" and also "fearful vocal affect". They also had problems processing "impending threat or punishment" Because of the difficulty processing emotions they have serious difficulties of learning from experience and this then leads them to repeat their behaviours. Blair (2004) has incorporated most of the low fear, low empathy positions into the new neuro-cognitive model, Integrated Emotion Systems model. Blair *et al* (2005) in discussing his Integrated Emotion System notes that "there is no single fear system but rather a series of at least partially separable neural systems that are engaged in specific forms of processing what can be subsumed under the umbrella fear". They also suggest there are "partially separable fear systems: for aversive conditioning/instrumental learning and for social threats (with this latter system in responding particularly to angry expressions" There is often obliviousness to fear in boys with psychopathic tendencies. Persons with Criminal Autistic Psychopathy tend to be fearless. Psychological and linguistic factors are shown in **Table 2**.

Table 2. Psychological and Linguistic factors

Psychological and Linguistic factors	Criminal Autistic Psychopathy	General psychopathy
Reduced reaction to upset in another person	Yes.	Yes.
Violence inhibition mechanism	Yes.(Criminal) Autistic Psychopathy.	Yes.
Reduced empathy	Yes.	Yes.
Theory of mind problems	Yes.	No.
Problems decentering self	Yes.	Yes.
Reduced observing self, mindfulness, self awareness	Yes.	Yes.
Reduced mentalising capacity	Yes.	Yes.
Emotion detection problems	Yes.	Probably.
Good systematising ability	Yes.	Yes.
Poor social reciprocity	Yes.	Yes.
Novelty seeking, sensation seeking	Autistic Psychopathy (Sometimes) Criminal Autistic Psychopathy.Yes.	Yes.
Fearlessness	Yes.Criminal Autistic Psychopathy.	Yes.
Emotional processing deficits	Yes.	Yes.
Moral deficits	Yes.	Yes.
Low affiliation	Yes.	Yes.
Low harm avoidance	Yes.	Yes.
Weak avoidance learning	Yes.	Yes.
Executive functioning deficits	Yes.	Yes.
Poor daily life management	Yes.	Yes (usually).
Pragmatic language problems	Yes.	Yes.

Mindfulness

Bishop *et al* (2004) operationally defined mindfulness as involving:

> "Self regulation of attention so that it is maintained on immediate experience, thereby allowing for increased recognition of mental events in the present moment".

It also involves "adopting a particular orientation towards ones experience in the present moment, or orientation that is characterised by curiosity, openness and acceptance". Persons with Autistic Psychopathy have problems paying attention in the general (other than things that they are interested in). They also have problems with set shifting and can get caught up in ruminative thinking. These would all be characteristic of poor mindfulness. Persons with Autistic Psychopathy would not show openness but would be defensive. They would also be deficient in mindfulness, which according to Bishop involves "gaining insight into the nature of one's mind and the adaptation of a de-centred perspective" They tend to be egocentric, often be only interested in concrete facts rather than being mindful of others subjectivity. Nevertheless in the Criminal Autistic Psychopathy subtype there is a deficiency of being mindful and empathic. Other characteristics of mindfulness according to Bishop (2004) include having an "observing self", "reflective functioning", "psychological mindedness", "self awareness", and having a decentred "perspective" Persons with Criminal Autistic Psychopathy would be deficient in all these areas (which really amount to good self awareness of others).

Sonderstrom (2003) correctly raises the issue of mentalising capacity in psychopathy. In psychopathy, Sonderstrom notes "the detached and stereotyped patterns of social interaction, semantic-pragmatic communication problems, poor ability to identity emotionally with others, to direct attention and to maintain central coherence" These factors are observed in serial killers and in Criminal Autistic Psychopathy.

Empathy

Adam Smith (1759) stated that:

> "as we have no immediate experience of what other men feel, we can form no idea of the manner in which they are affected, but by conceiving what we ourselves should feel in the like situation. Though our brother is upon the rack, as long as we ourselves are at our ease, our senses will never inform us what he suffers . . . it is by the imagination only that we can form any conception of what are his sensations". (in Woolf, 2001)

Nevertheless the non-psychopathic person can imagine to some extent the distress of the man on the rack. This kind of emotional imagination is deficient in General Psychopathy and Criminal Autistic Psychopathy. Smith was writing of course 250 years before the discovery of mirror neurons.

De Wied *et al* (2005) point out that "empathy is distinguished from sympathy and personal distress . . although the three constructs are closely related and often part of the same complex affective experience. Empathy involves a matching of emotions between the observer and target, i.e. feeling with another person. According to Eisenberg and colleagues (2000), empathy may turn into either sympathy (i.e. an other-oriented emotion), or personal distress (i.e. a self-focussed emotion), or some combination. Sympathy consists of feelings of sorrow or concern for the target, thus, feelings for another person. In contrast, personal distress is an aversive reaction, which may consist of feelings of discomfort or anxiety". This is not a feature of Criminal Autistic Psychopathy or General Psychopathy.

Hoffman (2000) points out that "empathy is the spark of human concern for others the glue that makes social life possible". Persons with General Psychopathy are not born with what Damasio (1994) calls "a neural propensity to generate somatic states with positive and negative emotions in response to environmental stimuli". Hoffman calls this the "affective change" which follows empathic behaviour. It is a core problem in psychopathy and Criminal Autistic Psychopathy.

Cooke and Michie (2001) noted that the deficient affective experience was associated with empathy deficits, fearlessness and lack of guilt with a tendency to blame others and make rationalisations. Kanner (1943) described autism as a disorder of "affective contact with people".

According to Baron-Cohen (2005), mind reading is defined as the ability to interpret one's own or another agent's actions as driven by mental states. Baron-Cohen's mind reading system focussed mostly on cognitive development. He has added in an affective component now which is clearly of critical importance and particularly critically important to the understanding of psychopathy. The component added he called TED or The Emotion Detector.

Baron-Cohen (2005) suggests that psychopathy may be associated with no difficulties in what he calls the "emotion detector" and no problems in the theory of mind mechanism but a problem in the empathising system. I have considerable doubts that it is so as clear-cut as this in the subgroup of Autism Spectrum Disorder/Criminal Autistic Psychopathy. He points out that:

> "the concept of mind reading itself I find too narrow, in that it makes no reference to the affective state in the observer triggered by recognition of another's mental state. This is a particular problem for any account of the distinction between autism and psychopathy. For this reason, the model is no longer of mind reading but of empathising and the revised model also includes a component TESS or the Empathising System".

The categories are never watertight but reflect a trend. Clearly this emphasising system is deficient in Criminal Autistic Psychopathy.

The mental problem in Criminal Autistic Psychopathy is low empathising. Persons with Criminal Autistic Psychopathy are not capable of reciprocity indeed are interested in precisely the opposite that is in control, domination, and degradation. These are all precisely the opposite to the capacity for empathising. The neural wiring for empathy is either absent or very malfunctioning in the person with Criminal Autistic Psychopathy. Of course the person with Criminal Autistic Psychopathy can still be very good at systematising, can be very good at mathematics, engineering, etc..

Persons with Criminal Autistic Psychopathy have not alone the extreme form of the male brain but the ultimate form of the male brain that is with minimal if not almost zero capacity for empathising. The idea of the serial killer as the ultimate form of the male brain in a negative sense is worth further examination. Criminal Autistic Psychopaths have a systematising style in their killing and have an identifiable style or modus operandi in how they go about it. It is quite possible that persons with Criminal Autistic Psychopathy who are serial killers have the lowest levels of empathising of any human being.

De Wied *et al* (2005) showed that boys with "disruptive behaviour disorders responded less empathically to sadness and anger" but normally to happiness. They also point out that "empathy may be viewed as a relatively stable disposition (dispositional empathy) but also as a transient affective reaction elicited in concrete situations (situational empathy)". De Wied *et al*'s findings were similar to those found by Cohen and Strayer (1996). Their study "demonstrated similar deficits in the dispositional and situational empathy among Conduct Disorder adolescents, and inverse relationships between both empathy measures and self-reported aggressive and socially maladjusted attitudes. Cohen and Strayer also provided evidence for greater deficits in emotion identification among Conduct Disorder youths as compared to normal controls". We are dealing here with a wide spectrum of antisocial behaviour and empathy deficits.

Blair *et al* (1996) note that "the capacity to empathise requires the ability to represent the mental states (the thoughts, the desires, hopes and feelings) of others. This ability has been referred to as "mentalising" or "theory of mind". Representations of the internal mental state of another person are assumed to act as stimuli for the activation of the affective, empathic response". If there is a problem in the empathy area it may be due to a problem with the capacity for mentalising or problems initiating and finding an empathic response. Blair *et al* (1996) did not find a theory of mind deficit in persons with psychopathy and concluded that the psychopath lacked the "emotional apparatus to feel empathy".

I believe that theory of mind deficit might be found in Criminal Autistic Psychopathy. It is not an all or none phenomenon. As Gillberg (1995) points out, you can get empathy deficit as well in persons with Attention Deficit Hyperactivity Disorder. Attention Deficit Hyperactivity Disorder is often associated with or antedates psychopathy. There are no clear boundaries between these conditions.

Peter Fonagy (2003) states that "when mentalisation fails, violence results". I believe he is quite right about this. Nevertheless this is not the cause of the violence of the serial killer with Criminal Autistic Psychopathy where it's the "thrill of the kill" which is often the driving factor.

Sonderstrom (2003) also notes that "the habitual lying in psychopathy is hardly comparable with good insight into other people's critical judgement and notorious "manipulation" is most often nothing but stereotyped and street mart attitudes that are rarely adjusted to situations requiring another type of display". It is often falsely believed that all persons with Autistic Psychopathy can't lie. Clearly the "social brain circuitry" is malfunctioning in all these conditions. Sonderstrom (2003) states that ASD is not "directly linked to cruelty, callousness, or dishonesty".

I am claiming in this book precisely the opposite that there is a subgroup of ASD (Autism Spectrum Disorder) which I call Criminal Autistic Psychopathy subtype where there is this capacity indeed the most extreme capacity of all human beings.

Fearlessness

A percentage of patients with Criminal Autistic Psychopathy subtype are fearless. Sonderstrom (2003) stated that this is because of their limited capacity "to visualise/imagine coming events" which diminishes their capacity to react appropriate to events. Cleckley (1976) stated that "within himself he appears almost incapable of anxiety as of profound remorse" Persons with Autistic Psychopathy in general show great anxiety and fearfulness but not in the subcategory of Criminal Autistic Psychopathy. Nevertheless I believe that persons with Criminal Autistic Psychopathy who are serial killers are well able to visualise the forthcoming killing process.

Newman (1998) pointed out that "whereas most people automatically anticipate the consequences of their actions, automatically feel shame for unkind deeds, automatically understand why they should persist in the face of frustration, automatically distrust propositions that seem to be good at the time, and are automatically aware of their commitments to others, psychopaths may only become aware of such factors with effort". This is also true for Autistic Psychopathy.

Indeed Lorenz and Newman (2002), note that "the impulsivity, poor passive avoidance, and emotional processing deficits of individuals with psychopathy may all be understood as a failure to process the meaning of information that is peripheral or incidental to their deliberate focus of attention" They have problems seeing the wider context. The same could be said of Criminal Autistic Psychopathy.

John Stone (2002) maintains that "the problem of autism has little to do with empathy, but involves an inability to understand complex social structures. Unsympathetic people, on the other hand, are often quite adept at manipulating such structures to their own ends and may often be (morally) criminal". I could not agree about autism having little to do with empathy.

But I agree with the problem of understanding social structures in criminality. They sometimes use psychology books to work out these structures.

Fearlessness is a feature of psychopathy and a subgroup of persons with Asperger's syndrome called Criminal Autistic Psychopathy. There is also a Behavioural Inhibition System (BIS) hypothesis about psychopathy, which emphasises weak behavioural inhibition. There is also the lack of impact of punishment on these persons, the inability to learn from experience, and problems with conditioning or being conditioned to societies norms (Fowles and Dindo, 2006).

Empathy and Blade Runner

Lauffer (2004) discusses Blade Runner a film adaptation of Philip Dick's (1963) novel *Do Androids Dream of Electric Sheep?* The drama takes place after a nuclear holocaust. Humans are in great distress and at risk of "dementation" and encouraged to emigrate to another planet and have an "android as a personal servant" These androids are very strong and intelligent but lack empathy (Lauffer, 2004). In the story, Dick (1982) describes an interaction with an android:

"the protagonist notes that . . . 'she smiled innocuously – at variance with (the stress serious implication of) her words . . . an android trait, possibly, he thought. No emotional awareness, no feeling-sense of the actual meaning of what she said. Only the hollow, formal, intellectual definitions of the separate terms. Another character senses, a peculiar and malign abstractness . . . in the android's mental processes."

Lauffer (2004) offers us here a parallel "between the clinical and the fictional". This gives a flavour of the person with Autistic Psychopathy and 'malignant tractness', the flavour of Criminal Autistic Psychopathy – the robotic type person.

Primary Psychopathy (Type 1)

It appears that the primary psychopath (Type 1 Psychopathy) has low arousal and needs thrill-seeking behaviour to deal with boredom, to cope with the unpleasantness of boredom by stimulus seeking behaviour, e.g. criminality or indeed serial killing. They have problems learning and attuning to societal values, to human values and to accepted morality. They have a largely egocentric narcissistic and self-interested points of view. Their self-concept is that of a killer for satisfaction, which they feel very comfortable with and can feel very relaxed afterwards. One of their multiple selves or self-concepts or identities is the killing self which is often the truest and most authentic sense of self that they feel.

Nigg (2006) describes Type 1 Psychopathy as being characterised by callous and unemotional traits. This type has high genetic input and low environmental input. Nigg also notes an association between Type 1 Psychopathy and temperamental low anxiety / low fear" as well as low "harm avoidance" and "weak avoidance learning" and "deficits in emotional processing and conditioning" and "low affiliation".

Lynam (2002) suggested that "the 'fledgling psychopath' was characterised by low affiliation, low conscientiousness (here, effortful or reactive control), and low negative affect (withdrawal)".

In understanding Criminal Autistic Psychopathy there is an increased emphasis on affective components over cognitive components. L. Kanner (1943) saw autism as a disturbance of affective relationships. Criminal Autistic Psychopathy is on an Autistic Spectrum and also on a General Psychopathic Spectrum.

Secondary Psychopathy (Type 2)

Nigg (2006) describes Type 2 psychopathy as showing reactive externalising and antisocial characteristics. Environmental factors are very important here and genetic factors play a minor role.

Blackburn (2006) notes that "introverts form anxiety responses more readily because they are more susceptible to fear or punishment cues". Secondary psychopaths suffer from more anxieties.

Frick and Marsee (20060 note a theory of psychopathy, which emphasises: "a deficit in the experience of certain emotions that guide pro-social behaviour and inhibit deviants."

Blackburn (2006) points out that "highly impulsive – low anxious offenders appear to correspond to primary psychopaths, impulsive – highly anxious offenders to secondary psychopaths. This implies that primary psychopaths have an over reactive BAS (Behavioural Activation System) and under reactive BIS (Behavioural Inhibition System), while in secondary psychopaths, both systems will be overactive" Blackburn discusses psychopathy as developmental delay. This is very interesting because Criminal Autistic Psychopathy is seen as a developmental disorder (Patrick 2006).

COGNITIVE ASPECTS OF PSYCHOPATHY

Frick and Marsee (2006) note another theory of psychopathy describing it as: "a cognitive deficit involving the ability of the person with psychopathy to use contextual cues that are peripheral to a dominant response set to modulate his or her behaviour.

Checkley (1976) notes psychopaths have "excellent rational powers (and) . . in full possession of his rational faculties". Mosby notes that Pinel (1801 – 1962) uses the phrase for psychopathy *manie sans delire* ("madness without confusion"). Pinel is referring to non-psychotic mental illness.

According to Hiatt and Newman (2006) there is also information processing deficits in psychopathy. These are the cognitive deficits. "Indeed psychopaths are notorious for the contrast between their good explicit knowledge and their profound failures when put to the test of daily life".

This can also go for Criminal Autistic Psychopathy. Hare (1986) noted that psychopaths "may not be able to focus attention on things of immediate interest, effectively ignoring warning cues and other stimuli not of immediate interest to them". Hiatt and Newman (2006) point out that "consistent with this proposal, many studies indicate that psychopaths fail to accommodate secondary or unattended information". This is context and fits with Criminal Autistic Psychopathy. They have this split between cognitive and emotional. They are narrow focussed on what is cognitively of interest to them and ignore the wider emotional context. They have the capacity to hyper focus on what is of interest to them. This suggests they have problems with attention shifting.

PSYCHOANALYTIC UNDERSTANDING OF CRIMINALS

Klein (1980) stated that "love is not absent in the criminal, but it is hidden and buried in such a way that nothing but analysis can bring it to light". This does not explain the Criminal Autistic Psychopathy or General Psychopathy.

The alternative psychoanalytic explanation is that the killer projects this murderous impulses, into the victim and then kills the victim, as a way of getting rid of these impulses. This does not explain Criminal Autistic Psychopathy who or the serial killer. Indeed nothing could be further from the truth.

EXECUTIVE FUNCTIONING (EF) PSYCHOPATHY AND CRIMINAL AUTISTIC PSYCHOPATHY

As Hill and Frith (2003) point out, executive function problems have been shown to be associated with autism indeed they show "poor daily life management" Executive function includes planning, working memory, impulse control, shifting from one task to another, inhibiting a prepotent response and perseveration. They are also associated with frontal lobe brain problems

Serial killers have problems in many of these areas. Executive dysfunction also occurs in General Psychopathy. Serial killers show poor life management.

Persons with Criminal Autistic Psychopathy remain focussed on some maladaptive way of functioning they cannot shift to a new perspective and they get stuck in this maladaptive over focussed pattern. They have difficulty seeing the big picture. This has a dehumanising effect and aids killing behaviour. See the overlap between Criminal Autistic Psychopathy and Attention Deficit Hyperactivity Disorder.

Geurts *et al* (2004). stated that:

> "ADHD was associated with Executive Function (EF) deficits in inhibiting a prepotent response and verbal fluency. The High Functioning Autism (HFA) group showed more difficulties than the ADHD group with planning and cognitive flexibility . . (the) HFA exhibit more generalised and profound problems with EF tasks compared to children with ADHD".

They also point out that "both ADHD and autism are categorised by behaviour similar to that found in patients with frontal lobe damage . . (and) neural imaging studies show involvement of prefrontal and connected structures in both ADHD and autism". "Poor behavioural inhibition is the central deficiency in ADHD and indeed psychopathy".

Geurts *et al* further point out that "Executive Function deficits are postulated as being the core cause in both ADHD and autism."

> "Compared to children with ADHD, the HFA group showed more difficulties with cognitive flexibility and planning. The deficits in cognitive flexibility for children with HFA might be related to the stereotyped repetitive patterns of behaviour that are characteristic for autism but not for ADHD. The present findings indicate that it is difficult to differentiate children with ADHD and children with HFA on the EF measures used here, although there are differences in both quantity and quality of the EF deficits across groups."

To fully understand Criminal Autistic Psychopathy and serial killing, the investigation needs to explore not only the autistic psychopathy but also the not uncommon overlap with Attention Deficit Hyperactivity Disorder. The combination diagnosis has a far greater explanatory power than a single diagnosis.

ADHD is commonly associated with Criminal Autistic Psychopathy and General Psychopathy.

Chapter 7

BRAIN/PSYCHOPATHY/AUTISTIC PSYCHOPATHY

Colin Blakemore (1988) stated that "our brain, our mind machine governs every human thought and action."

The brain is a tremendously complex organ with more than 10 billion neurons in a highly interconnected web governed by complex biochemical pathway – the most complex organ by far in the human body. It is hardly surprising that there is much that can go wrong with it.

Morrison (2005) points out that "scientists estimate that there are 300 million feet of wiring in the brain".

Beitman and Nair (2004) note "the phylogenetic path to the brain, with its ten billion neurons and an estimated $^{10}/_{15}$ synaptic connections".

Casanova (2005) also points out that "the human brain has anywhere from 50 to a couple of hundred different brain regions depending on the technique employed. Some of these areas seem to act independently from similar regions in the opposing hemisphere".

Hyman 2002 states that "real predictive power will come not from studying the 20 alleles in aggregate that give you a 30% risk of being somewhat more aggressive than the next guy; it will come from studying the nervous system" This chapter focuses on the nervous system.

MINICOLUMNS, ABNORMAL NEURAL CIRCUITRY, CREATIVITY, AND AUTISTIC PSYCHOPATHY

Minicolumns are the smallest brain models "traceable for processing information" according to Casanova (2005). Minicolumns are composed of both cells (neurons) and their projections that aggregate into standardised circuits. Recent studies suggest that minicolumns may be abnormal in autism. More specifically the brains of autistic patients have minicolumns that are smaller and more numerous than normal. Furthermore the cells (neurons) within each minicolumn are reduced in size. Since the metabolic efficiency of neuronal connectivity is a function of cell size, the presence of smaller neurons in the brains of autistic patients has a dramatic effect in the way that different parts of the brain interact with each other. Functions that require longer projections (e.g. language) may be impaired while shorter ones (e.g. mathematical manipulations) may be preserved or reinforced" This may partially explain the great creativity and savant talent seen in Autistic Psychopathy but also the less integrated brain, the brain with poor capacity for empathy. It is possible that empathy requires longer neural connections in the brain the ones that are impaired in Autistic Psychopathy with consequent major social interaction deficits.

This abnormal connectivity in the brain which makes the individual more 'robotic' and possessing less of the normal human empathic characteristics. It may be that this reduced neural connectivity allows certain areas of the brain to function more independently and therefore not be distracted by the "noise of normal human interpersonal relationships". These persons can then hyperfocus on certain topics. It is possible that this is happening in the brains of Criminal Autistic Psychopathy. Their hyperfocus is on killing or arson, etc..

According to Casanova (2005): "Minicolumns therefore account for the largest increase in brain size (as compared to overall body size) comparing humans to other species". "The total number of minicolumns is defined during the first 40 days of foetal development". There are problems with intrauterine neural circuitry development during this time, including problems in cell migration.

Casanova further states that "the small cell bodies of the brains of autistic patients favour information processing through short intra regional pathways, e.g. mathematical calculations, visual processing. Similarly cognitive functions that require long inter regional connections would provide metabolically sufficient, e.g. language, face recognition, joint retention.

INTUITION, AUTISM, AND VON ECONOMO NEURONS

Allman *et al* (2005) point out that "the Von Economo Neurons (VENs) are large bipolar cells located in layer 5 of the anterior cingulate (ACC) and fronto-insular (FI) cortex". They have emerged in the brain during the past 15 million years. Because of relatively recent onset they may be "particularly vulnerable to dysfunction". They appear at the "35th week of gestation" and less than 20% are present at birth but there is a full complement during the child's fourth year.

Allman *et al* (2005) hypothesise that problems with the development of VENs (Von Economo Neurons) are partially responsible for autistic social disabilities. VENs are necessary for "quick intuitive decisions" a major problem area in autism. This is important because Klin and Volkmar (1997) observed that "individuals with Asperger's Syndrome typically cannot avail themselves of their formal social knowledge in quick-paced, simultaneously shifting, social situations. They often miss the tempo of the interaction and lose any possibility of rapidly adjusting themselves to the forever shifting social and communicative demands of others.

Allman *et al* (2005) also point out the relevance of VENs to non-social uncertainty and quote Kanner as stating "the child's behaviour is governed by an anxiously obsessive desire for the maintenance of sameness. Changes in routine . . can drive him to despair". This is of critical importance.

Persons with theory of mind or understanding other minds are critical defects in Autistic Psychopathy and Criminal Autistic Psychopathy.

Allman *et al*'s (2005) hypothesis is that the VENs have a role "in the integration of the expectations of reward and punishment" and social relationships. Problems of brain integration are critical to Criminal Autistic Psychopathy.

Reduced brain interconnectivity is a key element of the problems in the autistic brain. The anterior cingulate and fronto-temporal cortex are also active when subjects experience guilt, embarrassment, and engage in deception. ACC and FI are also active in humour, trust, empathy, and the discrimination of mental states of others. One would expect abnormalities here in General Psychopathy and Criminal Autistic Psychopathy. These areas are involved in social relationships and there are vasopressin receptors in these areas as well. Vasopressin is involved in social behaviour in rodents and might be abnormal in psychopathy. Allman *et al* (2005) state that: "this right hemisphere VENs predominance may be related to the right hemispheric specialisation for the social emotions" which is disordered in Criminal Autistic Psychopathy.

Klin and Volkmar (1997) observed in Asperger's Syndrome "their deficient intuition and lack of spontaneous adaptation are accompanied by marked reliance on formalistic rules of behaviour and rigid social conventions" I hypothesise that there are problems in VEN in Criminal Autistic Psychopathy which will partially explain their social interactional problems.

THE FACE, BRAIN AND AUTISTIC PSYCHOPATHY

While issues in distributed neural networks now appear to be central to autism, that is problems of interconnectivity within the brain, there are also modular or more localised areas of abnormalities as well, i.e. the fusiform face area of the brain. According to Kanwisher (2006), "the fusiform face area, a blueberry-sized region on the bottom surface of the posterior right hemisphere that responds significantly more strongly when people look at faces".

Kanwisher (2006) points out that "highly specialised regions may be rare in the cortex" but do occur for example in relation to the face area. Nevertheless "the brain may also contain more general-purpose machinery that can operate across cognitive domains". The fusiform face needs specific resonance efforts in persons with General Psychopathy that is non-Autistic Psychopathy.

Fusiform gyrus abnormality seen in autism need to be studied extensively in General Psychopathy. This area is hypoactive in autism.

Persons with autism showed hypo-activation of the fusiform of the right fusiform gyrus in persons with autism. However, Pearse *et al* (2004) showed that this could be modulated depending on the familiarity and personal emotional content of the faces shown.

Ellis *et al* (1994) showed impairment in right hemisphere functioning in persons with Asperger's Syndrome as well as being "poorer at discriminating eye gaze and revealed difficulties in making hypothetical social judgements" Since the face is so fantastically important in social interaction it is hardly surprising that the brain gives it special attention. There are a vast number of facial expressions that have to be recognised. There is a major deficit here in Criminal Autistic Psychopathy.

Wickelgri (2005) stated that research using fMRI testing of "the ability to remember faces, there was varied connectivity abnormalities. In the autistic brains, links were weak between the front of the brain and the parietal lobe, between frontal regions and posterior perceptual brain areas, and between the face-processing brain region and other areas".

Wickelgri quotes an autism researcher as stating that "in study after study, we see a lower degree of synchronization in autistic brains". Wickelgri also stated that "the results suggest that neural circuits for action plans may not be fully intact in autism". This emphasises the interconnectivity problem in the brain that one would expect in Criminal Autistic Psychopathy.

Brain Grey and White Matter

Vlakeslee (2005) points out that white matter in the autistic brain is asymmetrical. She also points out that "white matter contains fibres that connect neurons in separate areas of the brain, whereas grey matter contains the neurons themselves".

Ectopic grey matter, that is grey matter in the wrong place, has also been shown in autistic brains by Bailey *et al* (1998).

Ellis *et al* (1994) pointed out that Semrud-Clickeman and Hynd (1990) suggested that in non-verbal learning disability which is very similar to Autistic Psychopathy that "there is a lesion or malfunction in white matter which has greater impact upon right hemisphere functioning because it has a greater dependence, for example, on callosal communication for intermodal integration of novel stimuli" Rourke (1988) noted a reduced white matter functioning in non-verbal learning disability.

In a study of pathological liars Yang *et al* (2005) showed that "it is possible that increased prefrontal white matter found in adult liars predisposes to lying" and that "reduction in prefrontal grey matter relative to white may be predisposed to a general antisocial disinhibition tendency" which has "implications for psychopathy". Of course there are probably many different pathways by which psychopathy develops. Yang *et al* (2005) showed that liars showed a 22 – 26% increase in prefrontal white matter and a 36 – 42% reduction in prefrontal grey / white ratios compared with both antisocial controls and normal controls.

In Autistic Psychopathy, research has shown 36% increase in white matter in the prefrontal lobes in autism and 22% in the occipital lobe at the posterior part of the brain. The differences are especially in parts of the brain that "integrate different types of information" Wickelgri (2005). These problems occur closer to the surface on the cortex. Local mental processing can be very good. To complicate matters, Eric Courchesne found the opposite that is "12% more grey matter" in the cortical areas of the brain in autism. When the frontal lobe is affected this leads to problems integrating different types of sensory information and problems with executive mental functioning including attention, planning and executing actions (Wickelgri, 2005). I would expect increased white matter in persons with Criminal Autistic Psychopathy.

Research on persons with Criminal Autistic Psychopathy has shown reduced levels of grey matter in the prefrontal cortical area of the brain. Research has also shown increased levels of white matter in the corpus callosum of persons with psychopathy which was associated with social relationship problems. Nancy Minshew *et al* (2005) noted that research showing the corpus callosum in persons with autism having reduced "white matter concentration" in the corpus callosum. The contradictory findings require further research with the possibility of subtyping resolving the contradictions.

Brain Size

Larger brain size is commonly discussed in relation to autism. It has been suggested as being due to inadequate pruning of neurons during development. According to Wickelgri (2005), Eric Courchesne suggests that "abnormal brain growth in autism occurs from birth to age three years".

Eric Courchesne described infants postnatally who later received a diagnosis of autism to have reduced head size at this point. This was followed by a 31 – 12 day growth spurt with additional accelerated growth between six months and 24 months. This accounts for the increased brain size. These events according to research worker Ruth Carper from Eric Courchesne lab particularly occur in the frontal cortex of the brain with very numerous nerve cells that are abnormal in size (Vlakeslee, 2005). These are problems in the frontal cortex in General Psychopathy and Criminal Autistic Psychopathy.

NEUROPATHOLOGY OF AUTISM AND PSYCHOPATHY

Pickett *et al* (2005) point out that the brain pathology studies in autism show "increased cell packing in the limbic system, reduced numbers of Purkinje cells in the cerebellum, and increased brain size, especially in the young autistic child, as measured by head circumference, MRI brain volume, and post-mortem brain weight" . Only a small proportion of these develop Criminal Autistic Psychopathy.

Raine and Yang (2002), in reviewing research on the Neuroanatomical Bases of Psychopathy, noted: (1) a larger corpus callosum, (2) a reduced volume of the posterior hippocampus, (3) diminished grey matter in the prefrontal cortex, and (4) reduction in the volume of the amygdala. Again one observes widespread abnormalities throughout the brain just like in Autistic Psychopathy.

BRAIN, AUTISTIC PSYCHOPATHY AND CONNECTIVITY

In autism there is under and over connectivity in the brain. Wickelgri (2005) notes that many autism researchers believe that autism results from abnormal communications between brain regions rather than a 'broken' part of the brain. She points out that one of the issues now is how do abnormal genes "perturb the development of neural connections" There is too much asynchrony in the brains of persons with autism. There is poor interpersonal connection in autism and poor connections between regions of the brain. Nevertheless, Wickelgri (2005) quotes the autism researcher Geraldine Dawson as stating that the connectivity issue might be "an effect – rather than a cause of an earlier dysfunction in the brain, such as a defect in brain systems that govern social reward."

Frontal Lobe, Autistic Psychopathy, and General Psychopathy

The frontal lobe occupies almost half of cortical space. Thompson (2006) quotes Professor Ian Robertson as stating "the brain is the most complex entity we know". "The frontal lobes of the brain – which are responsible for planning, forethought, controlling impulses, organisation and self-awareness – were the last part of the brain to be developed in evolution. They are also the last part to develop as we grow up. In humans, the frontal lobes are almost one-third of the brain, but in non-human primates, they are much smaller".

Frontal lobe functioning makes us moral and rational human beings. It is involved in fear conditioning and the socialisation of children and empathy. It is a kind of 'God-centre' of the brain. It contains our conscience. Our sense of self is organised in the frontal lobe (Lenzen, 2005).

Raine *et al* noted that "90 – 95% of the variance in prefrontal volume is determined by genetic factors". He also notes that it is likely that genetic factors play some role "in producing the type of structural prefrontal grey matter deficits previously found in psychopathic behaviour".

Damasio also said "to have a broader self, such as we do, requires an autobiographical memory" This is deficient in persons with Autistic Psychopathy leading to identity diffusion and a disturbed sense of self. The frontal lobe is critical to our sense of identity and sense of self.

The frontal lobe is the executive functioning centre of the brain as well as being involved in arousal and inhibition. It is the major control centre of the brain and is very widely connected to other centres of the brain. It is a major integrative centre of the brain. It is the planning centre of the brain. It is the major decision making centre of the brain. Its what makes us civilised people capable of forethought and not just impulsive animals.

Goldberg (2001) states that the frontal lobes "are the most uniquely human of all brain structures".

Raine (2002) points out that it "is likely that this prefrontal development has allowed humans to develop a social system that emphasises close cooperation, reciprocal altruism, and close living in groups" from an evolutionary point of view. This is a way of controlling aggression.

Blair *et al* (2006) state that lesions in the areas are associated with aggression. They also point out that "orbital and ventrolateral frontal cortex regulate the neural systems (the amygdala, hypothalamus and peri-aqueductal grey) that mediate the basic response to threat (including reactive aggression)".

Blair and Cipolotti (2000) hypothesised that "the neurons in the orbital frontal cortex are recruited by a system (termed social response reversal system) that is crucial for social cognition and modulation of reactive aggression".

Patients with frontal lobe problems tend to be more aggressive. The frontal lobes are associated with cognitive and socio-emotional processing. Raine *et al* (1992), in a study of murderers, found reduced glucose metabolism in both superior and inferior mesial frontal cortex and a trend towards reduction in orbital frontal cortex.

Murphy *et al* showed in ASD (Autism Spectrum Disorder) the "significant abnormalities in prefrontal lobe neural integrity, and this is related to severity of clinical symptoms". Wolff (2001) noted that "Damasio's theory is based on the discovery of a neural basis for pro-social behaviour, which is drastically impaired after damage to the prefrontal lobes".

Mentalising that is thinking about other people's mental states involves parts of the frontal and temporal cortex. These areas appear to be malfunctioning in General Psychopathy and Criminal Autistic Psychopathy. Abnormality in the frontal cortex also leads to problems in recognising fearful expressions on faces. This leads to a reduced capacity for interpersonal relating and in inhibiting aggression. Toal *et al* (2005) has shown "decreased activation of medial prefrontal cortex and amygdala during mentalising tasks in autism".

Rogers (2005) states that "it remains entirely possible that the emotional shallowness and interpersonal style characteristics of Clekley psychopathy are mediated by dysfunction in the dorsal medial and ventral prefrontal cortex sectors". "Failure to activate this shift of attention means that psychopaths are not able to interrupt maladaptive behaviour and regulate ongoing behaviour" Problems with attention shifting are also seen in Criminal Autistic Psychopathy which means that they carry on with the process of killing.

Moir and Jessel (1995) point out that in the frontal lobes "where the conscience abides, as well as temporal lobe abnormalities where damage, as we know, is associated with sexual deviancy. There was also low activity in the area of the limbic system which subserves memory and the frontal lobe – similar, though not identical, to the disconnection we have often observed within these two areas in psychopaths". They also point out in terms of sadistic killers a pattern "that researchers would associate with the damaged and sexually deviant mind, coupled with the frontal brain damage and resultant lack of conventional conscience".

Amygdala

Amygdala functioning is abnormal in Psychopathy and Criminal Autistic Psychopathy. The amygdala is part of the limbic system which also includes the hippocampal formation, olfactory regions and hypothalamus. The amygdala is involved in emotional experience and reactions and has 13 anatomically distinct nuclei. If the amygdala is damaged the person is then poor at recognising information from faces and voices. The amygdala is part of the limbic circuit with the anterior cingulate gyrus, ventro medial prefrontal cortex, ventral striatum and dosomedial nucleus of the thalamus. Its functions relate to motivation and emotional processing (Alexander *et al*, 1990).

In discussing the limbic system, Tancredi (2005) describes the amygdala as "the guard dog", the hippocampus as the "governor", the anterior cingulate cortex as the "mediator", and the hypothalamus as being involved in "master regulation".

Segal *et al* (2005) point out that "the amygdala processes the primitive emotions of fear, hate, love, and anger – all neighbours in the deep limbic brain we inherited from animals that evolved earlier. The amygdala works together with other brain centres that feed it or respond to it" Unfortunately the amygdala is not processing well in psychopathy or autism. The amygdala is involved in the emotional processing of other people.

Dobbs (2006) points out that Ralph Adolphs who is "an expert on emotion, memory and social cognition, has put it that the amygdala pervades the organisation of thought and behaviour at higher levels". Socially for instance according to Dobbs "patients with amygdala damage often overlook emotionally latent stimuli. They are slightly . . naïve". This is a feature of Criminal Autistic Psychopathy. "Growing evidence indicates that the amygdala enhances and directs our perception and attention regarding emotions other than fear, such as pleasure or disgust". Clearly this is a problem in Autistic Psychopathy of serial killers where they lack disgust when they cut up bodies etc. Dobbs also points out that "the amygdala helps to give life meaning. One implication is that the amygdala may play a leading role in establishing what consciousness researchers call salience – choosing which stimuli we prioritise and therefore what we are conscious" Salience for a serial killer is seeing a person who would make a suitable victim for killing.

Philips (2003) points out that many of these regions are involved in the "identification and response to emotionally salient information" and there are abnormalities in autism and psychopathy As Philips (2003) points out in relation to the amygdale, it is involved in face and eye gaze identification, emotional expression portrayed by others e.g. fear and auditory unpleasant stimuli.

Le Doux (2002) describes two pathways of emotional processing. In the first the emotional stimulus goes to the sensory thalamus and then directly to the amygdala from which an emotional response emanates. This is a "quick and dirty" method of emotional processing. It has echoes of how persons with psychopathy process emotional stimuli. The thalamus is a part of the brain that receives sensory impulses. "It is also the centre for the appreciation of primitive uncritical sensations of pain, crude touch" (Taber, 1965). A much more accurate but slower method of processing emotional stimuli is via the sensory thalamus onto the sensory cortex and then to the amygdala, which leads to a thought out emotional response, as well as dealing with emotional memories, and sets Dopamine pathway activation in association with past pleasurable memories which in relation to the serial killer would involve emotional memories of killing and a wish to kill more.

Lenzen (2005) points out that "feelings are what arise as the brain interprets emotions, which are themselves purely physical signals of the body reacting to external stimuli". He quotes Damasio telling him that feelings are not just the shady side of reason but that they help us to reach decisions as well. Damasio also stated that "when we feel sympathy for a sick person, we re-create that persons pain to a certain degree internally" Persons with Criminal Autistic Psychopathy might be aware of the person's pain intellectually but not emotionally. They have this separation between affect and intellectual processing.

Blair et al (2006) note that there is diminished amygdala "activation during emotional memory and aversive conditioning tasks" in psychopathy. They also have difficulties recognising fear on people's faces. This reduced the ability to become morally socialised. They tend to achieve their ends via aggressive behaviour. They are unresponsive to parenting skills therapy. Unfortunately naive Family Therapists think that they can cure psychopathy with Family Therapy.

Viding (2004) points out that "poor Violence Inhibitions Mechanisms (VIM) functioning and reduced sensitivity to punishment has been attributed to a sub-optimally operating amygdala at the neural level" It is possible that emotional processing by the amygdala is regulated by the prefrontal cortex and Le Doux (2002) suggests that "the amygdala may influence decision making and other cognitive functions of the prefrontal cortex" This is all relevant to the understanding of psychopathy. The amygdala has also a role in terms of assessing who might be a "sexually receptive" partner. In post-mortems studies in autism, Kemper and Bauman (1998) found abnormalities of size, density and dendritic arborisation in the amygdala. It would be illuminating to study the post-mortem amygdala of serial killers.

Moir and Jessel (1995) point out that in criminality "the right side of the amygdala seems overactive".

The amygdala shows abnormal development in autism as noted by Pickett (2005). Pickett and London noted that "with an antemorten MRI, they found the amygdala in autistic boys was adult size by approximately 8 years of age and did not enlarge as compared with typically developing male children who show a protracted increase in volume, reaching an adult size in late adolescence". They stated that "the entire amygdala including its lateral nucleus, had significantly fewer neurons in autistic brains compared with each matched controls, particularly in adults".

There is very clear genetic input into psychopathy and therefore amygdala dysfunction. This impairment in the functioning of the nerve cells of the amygdala leads to impaired emotional processing and learning which leads to aggression and antisocial behaviour as well as diminished recognition of fear on faces as well as superego or conscience deficits and reduced capacity for empathy.

In addition, Blair *et al* (2006) point out that amygdala dysfunction "disrupts the ability of the individual to be socialized and thus puts them at greater risk of learning antisocial behaviours, including instrumental aggression, to achieve their goals".

According to Blair *et al* (2005) "socialisation involves aversive conditioning and instrumental learning" A malfunctioning amygdala interferes with both these processes and leads to an unsocialised child. Persons with psychopathy have problems learning from experience. Proper superego/conscience development requires an individual to be aware that they are hurting another individual and then to develop a sense of guilt about this. This is a major problem in psychopathy because of the malfunctioning amygdala. They are not good at processing good emotional experiences either although they have a much greater deficit in processing negative emotional experiences. Persons with psychopathy have less problems in processing eye emotion than persons with classic autism. Of course in this book, we are focussing on a subcategory of ASD Autism Spectrum Disorder Criminal Autistic Psychopathy subtype. Therefore amygdala and frontal lobe malfunctioning is important in psychopathy. The amygdala is also hypoactive in facial perception tasks in Autistic Psychopathy.

Sonderstrom (2003) states that problems in the amygdala leads to fearlessness, empathy difficulties, problems with social cognition and reading of emotions.

Moir and Jessel (1995) note that the amygdala is abnormal in "sexual sadists".

Persons with psychopathy have problems learning from positive or negative experiences in their environment. They are stuck in old maladaptive, primitive patterns of behaviour. They use violence at times rather than rational persuasion to achieve their ends. It is as if they are at times "shutting out the cerebral cortex". They are often too impatient impulsive for subtle rational logical persuasion.

In discussing ASDs, Blair *et al* (2005) state that in comparison to psychopathy there "are gross differences in disorder". I am presenting the opposite view in this book and showing that in Criminal Autistic Psychopathy subtype there are great overlapping features. There is no sharp dividing line between psychopathy/Autistic Psychopathy and Attention Deficit Hyperactivity Disorder. Genes can have multiple effects and these could be some similar genes underlying all three conditions. All conditions have frontal lobe problems and executive function problems albeit with some variability between them. Nevertheless, there is massive heterogeneity and overlap in many so-called independent categorical disorders. Persons with autism and psychopathy show clear empathy deficits and empathy deficits are also not uncommon in Attention Deficit Hyperactivity Disorder.

A full psychiatric assessment in forensic patients should have dimensional assessment of the three disorders. Criminal Autistic Psychopathy and ADHD are very often missed in forensic populations. In autism the amygdala starts off having an increased size but in adults the "amygdala in autism is abnormally small" (Baron-Cohen et al 2005). At the same time in relation to amygdala size in autism the findings are contradictory – some show enlargement, others show a normal size, and another shows smaller amygdala values. Measurement error, diagnostic error and heterogeneity are probably relevant here.

Sonderstrom (2003) describes an fMRI study of "affective memory activation in psychopathy which showed decreased activation of the cingulate, ventral striatum, and amygdala / hippocampal formation, in combination with increased cortical activity in other fronto-temporal areas indicating non-limbic cognitive strategies to process affective words". Gillberg et al (2000) have shown that there are problems of callosal functioning in violent offenders. Baron-Cohen et al (1999) showed using fMRI that "patients with autism or Asperger's Syndrome activated the fronto-temporal regions but not the amygdala when making mentalistic inferences from the eyes" They are therefore using different parts of the brain to non-autistic persons as are persons with psychopathy and Criminal Autistic Psychopathy.

Insula and Anterior Cingulate

According to Beitman and Nair (2004): "The cingulate gyrus which is a multifunctional associative cortex, is essential for advanced self-awareness. Without cingulate function, the entire motivational dimension of the self will be non-functional. Individuals with cingulate damage are not aware that anything is missing because they lack the ability to assemble the higher order cortical maps that represents object value and provide the motivation for action"

Phillips (2003) also points out that the "anterior (agranular) insula" is also involved in negative stimuli and "fear reactivity".

Craig (2004) points out that there is evidence that "right anterior insula (rAI) is important for explicit subjective awareness and, significantly, offer a substantive anatomical explanation as to why some individuals are more aware of their feelings than others". He points out that "individual differences in subjective interceptive awareness, and by extension emotional depth and complexity, might be expressed in the degree of expansion of rAI and adjacent orbito-frontal cortices". He also points out that "a morphological correlation also exists between Alexithymia and the right anterior cingulate" It is interesting that Alexithymia and Autistic Psychopathy are often confused (Fitzgerald and Bellgrove, 2006). Alexithymia is often associated with hypochondriacal symptoms which also often occur in Autistic Psychopathy. Both of these patients have a poor sense of self and major problems expressing feelings.

Miller (2005) also reported that research had shown that an area of the brain called the insula was active when felt disgust either in themselves or in watching it in others. This reaction would appear to be impaired in psychopaths of the necrophilac variety and many serial killers.

The issue of a disturbance of a sense of disgust is critical to cannibalism. They have problems with self and other disgust. They are not inhibited by their disgusting behaviour. The interior insula may also be a brain inhibitory area.

According to Schore,

> "the right insula ... (is) involved in emotional and facial processing, in integrating tonal structures with a speakers emotions and attitudes . . . in pain processing (2003)"

It is interesting that both General Psychopathy and Criminal Autistic Psychopathy both have speech and language problems. The insula is also part of the limbic system which is disordered in these conditions and emotional processing of facial emotion is difficult in Criminal Autistic Psychopathy.

Temporal Lobe

Moir and Jessel (1995) state that "not only the sex-centres of the left temporal lobe, but also the aggression-control areas of the right – which we have already seen to be damaged in epileptics and in some sexual deviations such as paedophilia – showed abnormalities". "In sexual sadists there was specific damage to right temporal lobe – an area which is also responsible for the control of aggression".

Lavgevin (1991) showed that 40% of sex murderers had some abnormality in the right temporal horn of the brain.

Cerebral Lateralisation

Lalumiere *et al* (2001) stated that "psychopaths show less cerebral lateralisation than non-psychopaths". Paradoxically this is closer to the female pattern and it does not seem to help the brain in social processing. This might go with identity diffusion.

Some studies have shown "reverse or absent lateralisation of brain activity in autism" (Sigman *et al,* 1997). What one can conclude is that cerebral lateralisation is not normal in General Psychopathy and Autistic Psychopathy but more research is needed to get conclusive findings. Of course it would have been extraordinary if it had been normal. Again more careful subtyping might clarify the problem.

Autonomic Nervous System

Wolff (2001) notes that Damasio noted that "patients who had sustained prefrontal lobe damage in adult life did not have the usual autonomic nervous system responses to being shown fleeting pictures of cruelty and disasters, although they could remember clearly what they had seen. Retrospectively they indicated that the feelings of distress they would have had in response to the pictures prior to their injury were now lacking" (Damasio, 1994). This seems very important in General Psychopathy and probably in the autistic subgroup of Criminal Autistic Psychopathy.

Hirstein *et al* (2001) hypothesised that "autistic children use overt behaviour to control a malfunctioning autonomic nervous system". Whether this could be applied to psychopathy is not clear. Psychopathic behaviour is the best life solution these persons have been able to come up with.

Hirstein *et al* (2001) also noted that children with autism show mostly hyper-responsive activity of the sympathetic branch of the autonomic nervous system and a smaller very important group showed hyposensitive sympathetic activity. Extreme findings like this are very common in autism studies and again show the massive heterogeneity. We use the word autism but we are dealing with a group of conditions which share some common core characteristics but also many differences in presentations and neurobiological profiles.

Morrison *et al* (2004) point out that "many serial murders will complain or talk about being hypertensive or having multiple autonomic symptoms, from sweating to rapid heartbeat to vomiting to passing gas at the time or just prior to the act of killing" . Extremes of sensitivity reaction are common in autism i.e. hyper or hypo. Lalumiere *et al* (2001) point out that psychopaths are less physiologically reactive when exposed to cues of distress". In Criminal Autistic Psychopathy, you would expect low reactivity.

MALE: FEMALE BRAINS, GENDER AND PSYCHOPATHY

Autism and psychopathy are far commoner in males. Could this have something to do with differences in male and female brains? Cahill (2005) points out that "anatomical difference occurs in every lobe of male and female brains" Some areas are enlarged in females and others in males e.g. the amygdala is larger in men and the hippocampus is larger in women. Cahill (2005) noted that "the realisation that male and female brains were processing the same emotionally arousing material into memory differently led him to remember that there was a theory stating that the right hemisphere is biased towards processing the central aspects of a situation, whereas the left hemisphere tends to process the finer details" He showed that when Propranolol a drug that dampens the amygdala was given to men they were less able to process the central aspects of a situation or gist.

Cahill (2005) showed a slide of a decaying animal "men who reported strong responses showed greatest activity in the right hemisphere amygdala . . . whereas women who felt most worked up and showed the best recall displayed greatest activity in the left amygdala" They also pointed out that it was likely that "hemispheric sex differences in amygdala activity caused women to be more likely to retain details of an emotional event and men are more likely to remember its gist" There have been old studies showing higher Serotonin levels in some persons with autism than controls in the blood. Females have a more integrated less lateralised brain and they are more empathic, more sensitive, have better verbal skills, and are better at emotional processing, have less Attention Deficit Hyperactivity Disorder autism and psychopathy. Cahill (2005) also pointed out that they may be better at stress management than males and "it is still unclear . . . what protects female hippocampal cells from the damaging effects of chronic stress, but sex hormones are likely to play a role" If the brain is less damaged by stress in females this might partially explain some of the sex differences in psychiatric disorders.

Lloyd (2006), in a report of neuroimaging study co-ordinated by Larry Cahill, stated that "throughout evolution, women have had to deal with a number of internal stressors, such as childbirth, that men haven't had to experience. What is fascinating about this is the brain seems to have evolved to be in tune with those different stressors". "The scans also showed that men's and women's amygdalas are polar opposites in terms of connections with other parts of the brain. In men, the right amygdala is more active and shows more connections with other brain regions. In women, the same is true of the left amygdala".

Hawkes (1995) points out that "by measuring the rate at which different parts of the brain burn glucose, a team from the university of Pennsylvania has concluded that men tend to be better at tasks requiring dexterity and good perception of space, while women are better at some verbal tasks and in those involving emotional judgement". "They found that in general similarities between men and women were greater than differences. But men showed a higher metabolic rate in the temporal limbic system of the brain, and women in a region called the cingulate gyrus".

"Anatomic differences in the brain have also been demonstrated. These differences include the size and shape of major fibre tracts that cross between the right and left hemispheres of the brain, such as the corpus callosum and the anterior commissure (which connects the temporal lobes), as well as regions of the brain including the prefrontal cortex. Such studies have shown that women have a larger corpus callosum – particularly the posterior portion – and anterior commissure than heterosexual men". Tancredi (2005) points out that "various nuclei of the medial amygdala are much larger in males than females". Their brains are more inter-connected.

There is increased white matter in male brain and a 9% increase in the cerebrum. There is evidence that the corpus callosum which connects the two cerebral hemispheres is smaller in men. Baron-Cohen *et al* (2005) point out that "there are more neurons in the male cerebral cortex, and in general, these neurons are more densely packed". They suggest that the findings suggest "increased local connectivity and decreased intra-hemispheric or (long range) connectivity in the male brain". The female brain is less lateralised and language shows more evidence in the female of bilaterality, "suggesting greater inter hemispheric connectivity" and a "single study of gamma-band magnetoencephalography report increased phase locking between frontal and parietal sites in women during cognitive performance, again suggesting greater long-range connectivity"

In larger brains which are not uncommon in autism there appears to be less interconnectivity of the brain which mean less long range integrated processing but more local processing which goes with being better at systematising. The parts of the male brain are less "joined up" giving less integrated brain, which may give a sense of multiple selves or identity diffusion which gives a poorer sense of self and other and therefore poorer capacity for communication. This may very well be exaggerated in the case in Criminal Autistic Psychopathy and General Psychopathy.

Baron-Cohen *et al* (2005) note that it is important to "distinguish brain dimorphisms mediated by testosterone and those that arise more directly from genetic factors or those that depend on experience". "Because 15% of x-chromosome genes escape x-inactivation in humans, x-chromosome gene-dosage affects may play a role in such direct genetic effects". They point out that "although males and females do not differ in general intelligence, specific cognitive tasks reveals sex differences". Skuse (2000) has suggested that an imprinted x-locus could explain sex differences in social and communicative skills and the male problems in social and communicated impairments.

Males are superior at map reading, like mechanical things, like cars, and are attracted to careers in engineering and computers – systematising careers. Females talk earlier and like doll play and career that focus on communication and require good empathy.

According to Sonnenmoser (2005), females are superior to males "in judging the character of others" and more empathic. They use their feelings more in decision making and rely more on "amygdala feeling". Females make more use of their "language centres". They have better verbal skills and more "emotional access to other people". They have less autism and psychopathy. These positive female abilities may give some protection against General Psychopathy and Criminal Autistic Psychopathy.

MIRROR NEURONS AND THE DEVELOPMENT OF THE BRAIN AND PSYCHOPATHOLOGY: MIRROR NEURONS AND MORALITY

Mirror neurons in the brain help children (and us) to learn by imitating other people's behaviour. They help us to imitate other people's moral behaviour. Of course they will also help people imitate immoral, sadistic, perverse behaviour whether in society or on television. According to Tancredi (2005), the mirror neurons "in humans involve a network, which is formed by the temporal, occipital, and parietal visual areas, as well as two additional cortical regions that are predominantly motor. These last two regions are the inferior parietal lobe (rostral part) and the precentral gyrus (lower part) and the posterior part of the inferior frontal gyrus. Together, these regions constitute the mirror neuron system in humans".

The *Dictionary of Biological Psychology* (2001) points out that the mirror neuron "in the cortex comes into action by the observation of an appropriate movement in another individual. It is thought that such events reveal important information about mental representations in the brain" Problems with mirror neuron functioning are probably important in Criminal Autistic Psychopathy and General Psychopathy.

Wickelgri (2005) quotes Miller as stating that "it appears that the mirror-neuron system is impaired in autism because the long fibre tracts that connect to the mirror neurons are not as well organised".

Miller (2005) gives an example of the action of the mirror neurons, using the tarantula scene from the James Bond film *Dr. No*. He states that "you get the creeps watching the spider crawl up James Bond's arm, it maybe because the scene fires up the same neurons that would be active were the spider making it up your arm" This mechanism is malfunctioning in Autistic Psychopathy and is probably malfunctioning as well in General Psychopathy and partially accounts for the lack of empathy, lack of disgust, and failure to tune in to the victims pain. Indeed it leads to dehumanisation of people or what psychoanalysts call part-object relationships. Mirror neurone pathology leads to problems "reading" other people and working out responses to them.

For most people, when witnessing a serial killer or a movie or reading about them do not imitate their actions, but nevertheless a predisposed individual could be precipitated into a copycat situation. People with this mirror neuron pathology will have difficulty picking up normal social behaviour from their observation of family and school life in childhood. They have problems learning from good experience and in learning empathic interpersonal ways of behaving. They have problems working out other people's motivations. They are significantly cut off in their own one person world and have major difficulty in relating to the multi-person world. Childhood prohibitions and sanction for deviant behaviour do not lead to change of behaviour in persons with General Psychopathy and Criminal Autistic Psychopathy.

NEUROETHICS, FREE WILL AND CRIME

Man has only a limited capacity for free will or choice in his actions. In ancient times man was felt to be controlled by the Gods and therefore free will did not come into it. Free will is limited by unconscious factors.

Churchland (2005) states that: "I don't think that the only time I am exercising free will is when I am agonising, but for all my in control behaviour. I am exercising free will right now when my words are coming out of my mouth, and I don't have any chance to deliberate. If I deliberate on my next utterance, then of course I get tongue-tied and I make a real hash of it". "The most fundamental neuroethical issue concerns free will and responsibility. The mind is what the brain does, and the brain is a causal machine. Consequently, deliberations, beliefs, decisions and ensuing behaviour are the outcome of causal processes. Typically the causal processes that lead to awareness of a decision are non-conscious" She points out that according to Gazzaniga (2005) "the brain is determined, but the person is free". I can't agree with this particularly in relation to Criminal Autistic Psychopathy where the person is so driven that they are not personally free and have a very unintegrated brain.

Wegner (2002) wrote a book called *The Illusion of Conscious Will* In truth, it is partly an illusion. While human behaviour is driven by neurobiological process, when we do something, we often make up a reason for doing it in retrospect. We are not in general free agents but serial killers are far less free than non-killers are. As well as biological processes including genes, various severe traumas in earlier life can operate unconsciously to decrease our free will. There is no doubt that the criminal justice system grossly exaggerates people's capacity for free will and fully blames people for actions that they were only partly responsible for at most. The criminal justice's systems view of the mind is grossly old fashioned and out of date – sometimes hundreds of years out of date. The use of the idea of precedence, or previous judgements has catastrophic negative effects in the legal judgements in the here and now in the mental health area. Precedence throws out modern science. Personal moral judgements are significantly influenced by nature or biology as well as environment or nurture. Charles Darwin with his evolutionary theory played a huge role in the emphasis on biology as did Sigmund Freud who was a Darwinian at times biology sets limits on our capacity to make good moral judgements. The limbic system which processes emotions and the prefrontal lobe or central control agency in the brain has huge effects on our capacity to make moral judgements. Testosterone affects our ability to make moral decisions.

Gazzaniga *et al* (2005) point out that "the link between the brain and behaviour is much closer than the link between genes and behaviour". "The brain determines the mind". "If the brain carries out its work before one becomes consciously aware of a thought, as most neuroscientists now accept its true, it would appear that the brain enables the mind". "If the readiness potential of the brain is initiated before we are aware of making the decision to move our hand, then it would appear that our brains know our decisions before we become conscious of them" This has an impact on criminal responsibility.

Hooke (2005) notes that Paul Churchland stated that "at least some failures of moral character, therefore, and especially the most serious failures, are likely to involve some confounding disability or marginality at the level of brain structure and/or physiological activity". I strongly agree with this.

Patricia Churchland (2005) points out that "badness, just as much as madness, involves the brain". She points out correctly that "it is precisely because an important difference exists between a normal brain and the brain of someone who is seriously demented or unreachably deluded that such people are not considered responsible for crimes they might commit" Persons with General Psychopathy and Criminal Autistic Psychopathy have diminished responsibility.

Chapter 8

EVIL AND ETHICS

Depue *et al* (2005) state that:

> "Evil is more than a vague notion. It is an entity, and it is manifest on the earth. It has reflexes and intuition, senses vulnerability and changes its form to adapt to its surroundings. Those who do not believe in the devil walk this earth have not seen the things that I have seen". He goes on to point out that Evil. . "is born in the mind, takes root there as fantasy, and prospers when normal human restraint no longer contains it."

I believe evil is rooted in genes and the environment.

According to Lenzen (2005): "Social feelings such as sympathy, shame or pride – they form a foundation for morality". Persons with Criminal Autistic Psychopathy are lacking these and thus are not surprisingly described as evil

A person with schizophrenia acting on a voice tells them to kill someone would not be committing an evil act. Valley (2004) describes evil as unfathomable and that "evil threatens human reason" and that "it challenges our hope that the world makes sense". He notes that "evil challenges our sense of order". In the past he pointed out that evil was "a form of "possession" by some outside devil". Harold Shipman shows how far we are from understanding evil. Evil had to be exorcised or banished in some way in the past.

Hansford (1967) points out that "I have also suggested that we all too readily comfort ourselves by believing there can be no such thing as wickedness: that there is only sickness – that is, a thing for which the subject bares no responsibility. I believe that some of us are, or can be, fairly wicked". Evil has a significant biological basis.

Evil appears to be a potentiality in everyone. Nevertheless, I do see Criminal Autistic Psychopathy of the serial killer as quite different from normality. It appears to me that people who engage in evil acts know intellectually what they are doing but not emotionally. According to Baumeister (1997): "the prototypes of human evil involve actions that intentionally harm other people. Defining evil as intentional interpersonal harm leaves many grey areas" Persons who are sexual predators are egocentric, narcissistic, and grandiose and lack empathy, features that are associated with persons who engage in evil acts. Evil is not a myth in my view.

In religious teaching evil is often associated with the seven deadly sins. Laqueur (2005) points out that:

> "Julia Kristeva once noted, medieval men and women would have found it easier to accept the notion of evil than modern man, including forensic scientists. Some of them at least, until recently, have regarded evil as an absurd notion for which there was no room in their discipline."

Psychiatrists and psychologists are 'phobic' of the word evil. From the biblical point of view evil started with Adam and Eve in the Garden of Eden. Evil is quite problematic for religious people. Evil is what serial killers do by and large.

Trakakis (2004) states that: "for if we assume that god must always chose the best, then our world must be, as Leibnitz infamously stated, the best of all possible worlds (or the best world creatable by god)". Trakakis notes the "evidential argument for evil. But if there were a god there would be no pointless suffering. Therefore it is highly unlikely that there is a god".

Baumeister (1997) points out that:

> "the great thinkers St. Thomas Aquinas wrote that the existence of evil in the world is the single greatest obstacle to Christian faith and doctrine. In other words, nothing undermines the Christian belief in god more than the existence of evil. If god is all good and all powerful, how can god allow evil to happen?"

Theologians have approached this problem through 'Theo-babble'. Of course, Aquinas is correct in this and we are not controlled by gods, but by our genes and environments. Hitler's willing executioners of the Jews show how close average persons (e.g. low ranking public servants) can be to perpetrating evil in a group situation or where it is sanctioned by higher authority.

St. Augustine stated "it is not we ourselves that sin, but some other nature sins in us". (St. Augustine's Confessions Book Five.) This again has the Jekyll and Hyde notion the split in one between good and evil in the personality between normal living and sinning or killing. Between god and the devil. St. Augustine was right about the nature of sin.

Masters (1993) talks about "Dionysian verges of . . destruction and anarchy, and they have to be kept in check by the structure of civilisation, including religion and morality . . in Dahlmer's case (a serial killer). . Dionysus broke lose". Masters notes that Dionysus was reputed to be "wild, instinctive, and dangerous". The same could be said of the serial killer who has Criminal Autistic Psychopathy. Civilisation is partly located in the frontal lobe of the brain, which is usually malfunctioning when a person commits an evil act.

Huxley (1982) went much too far when he identified human beings as primarily evil. It is true that men are often very egocentric and narcissistic and the history of man is a history of repeated genocide but that is only one side of man or some men. Civilisation progressed with the development of the frontal lobe, with conscience, and morally associated development. Innumerable genetic mutations and selective processes were critical in this evolution.

Thompson (2006) asked Professor Ian Robertson . a psychologist, the following question: What were his views on the evolution versus creationist issue, or science versus religion debate? "I don't think religion has anything to say about the physical world. Science has managed to explain the physical world extremely well. Religion has its own areas of responsibility, which are morals, ethics and offering people access to other realms of human consciousness. Religion and science can co-exist happily if they each stick to what they are good at".

Chapter 9

DOPAMINE OTHER NEUROCHEMICALS, HORMONES AND CROSS CULTURAL ISSUES

Dopamine is a brain neurochemical involved in salience, attention, and reward. According to Beitman and Nair (2004):

> "Objects and events lose individual importance, because they do not emerge from the perceptual background, and the organism has difficulty generating a motivational state related to the perceived objects. With too much Dopamine, the opposite occurs, and objects and events can be imbued with excessive salience"

In Autistic Psychopaths killing has excessive salience.

For example, Bundy when he saw women with their hair parted in the middle had increased salience. Whether serial killers need to take more risks as their killing career progresses to increase Dopamine levels to previous levels by increasing risk is not certain. Certainly they show increased carelessness which increases the risk of being caught.

Le Doux (2002) notes a hypothesis that:

> "Dopamine is involved in the switching of attention and selection of action."

It is possible that Dopamine is involved in the run up to a killing with serial killers and in the selection of victims.

> "Prefrontal cortex can exert an inhibitory influence on Dopaminergic release . . . through activation of inhibitory inter neurons. This provides a cortical modulation of limbically driven activities (look before you jump). The system can be overwhelmed, for practical purposes, by release of large amounts of Dopamine into the nucleus accumbens combined with at least one strong, reward-signalling cue. This promotes a limbic override of behaviour directions proposed by the cortex and amplification of reward seeking behaviours, and is an important component of drug addiction. The individual who falls into this state has difficulty shifting attention from the highly salient object or situation that caused the Dopamine release."

This seems to be the situation with serial killers. There are contradicting findings in the literature in relation to Dopamine.(Minzenberg and Siever, 2006).

Persons with psychopathy who are serial killers clearly find the activity rewarding. The neurochemical associated with reward is Dopamine. There is question whether Dopamine is involved when the serial killer anticipates a killing? If it was then a Dopamine blocking drug might have a role in psychopathy. There is some plausibility to this hypothesis. Certainly risk takers/sensation seekers have the Dopamine novelty seeking genetic polymorphism (DRD4) (Kirley et al, 2004).

C. Marsden (2006) conclude that:

"Dopamine neurons account for less than 1% of the neurons in the brain, but changes in the levels or functional state of brain Dopamine can have profound behavioural effects, suggesting that the role of Dopamine is not to relate specific information but to integrate information relevant to the incoming biologically important stimuli."

Autistic Psychopathy is a major disorder of poor integration of the brain.

MONAMINE OXIDASE (MAO)

There is evidence for an association between lower MAO activity and psychopathy, delinquency, impulsiveness, aggressiveness, poor socialisation, adult repetitive offending, and sensation seeking or novelty seeking. Nevertheless this requires much future research.

Monamine Oxidase (MAO) is involved in degrading the neurochemical Serotonin. Minzenberg and Siever (2006), noted that in relation to "psychopathy related symptoms" those persons with low MAO had "high impulsiveness, irritability, and low socialisation") and this was also seen in persons with "Checkley Psychopathy criteria". Persons with psychopathy often show sensation seeking characteristics and this is also associated with low MAO. Minzenberg et al note that: "a recent line of investigation suggests an intriguing link between Monoaminergic disturbances and a neurocognitive deficit that may underlie the social and emotional dysfunction that is a hallmark of psychopathy".

Churchland (2005) points out that the New Zealand longitudinal follow-up study, which showed "a significant subpopulation showed a strong and unmodifiable disposition to engage in antisocial behaviour, including irrational and self-destructive violence. Genetic analysis revealed that most of the men in that subpopulation carried a mutation for a particular enzyme Monamine oxidase (MAOA). The enzyme metabolises three neuromodulators (Serotonin, Norephrenine, and Dopamine all of which are relatively concentrated in the prefrontal areas of the cortex), thereby inactivating them. Those who had this mutation had an 85% chance of being involved in antisocial behaviour as compared to 22% who had not been maltreated" Clearly these factors (genetic and environmental) would have to be taken into account by courts. She also points out that the capacity of those with "the MAOA mutation to acquire an act on social norms appears to be diminished".

There is some evidence that those involved in sexually perverse behaviour and sensation seeking behaviour have these genetic abnormalities (Domschke et al, 2005). Attention Deficit Hyperactivity Disorder is associated with or antedates psychopathy and has also been associated with the Dopamine novelty seeking polymorphism (DRD4). (Kierley et al, 2004)

NORADRENALINE

Minzenberg and Siever (2006) point out that "lower levels of Noradrenaline in arrested men awaiting trial who scored above the median on a scale derived from Checkley criteria." Raine (2002) points out that "low resting heart rate is associated with aggressive behaviour and "may reflect reduced Noradrenergic functioning and a fearless, stimulation – seeking temperament". Certification of the Noradrenaline findings will require further research because of the contradictory findings. Distinct subgroups might be the expalantion of the contrdictatory findinsg. He also states that:

> "low arousal, stimulation seeking, fearlessness, increased vagal tone – vagal passive coping, reduced Noradrenergic functioning, and reduced right hemisphere functioning represent several of the possible processes which either by themselves or in combination may predispose a child to aggression."

He also goes on to state that "strong under arousal of the sympathetic nervous system would support a neurochemical explanation of the heart rate – antisocial relationship based on reduced Noradrenergic functioning" There is also evidence for "reduced heart rate and reduced Noradrenaline in conduct disordered children".

Siever (1998) points out that in impulsive personality: "increases in Noradrenergic responsiveness may be associated with greater engagement with and reactivity to the environment . . . such individuals having difficulties in suppressing aggressive behaviour, making it more likely that they will respond aggressively to any provocation".

Siever sees "Noradrenergic measures as being more closely linked to sensation seeking, risk taking, hostility, and irritability, whereas the Serotonergic measures are more closely correlated with direct physical manifestations of aggression".

Blum (1997) noted that unusually high levels of Noradrenaline have been found in a series of violent men. Very high levels of Noradrenaline are also found in people who attempt suicide in the bloodiest possible ways" She also points out that "vicious and violent experience sends Noradrenaline screaming upward".

Attention Deficit Hyperactivity Disorder has been shown to have Noradrenaline dysfunction like psychopathy and is often associated with psychopathy.

Raine (2002) notes that the effects of:

> "smoking exposure on Noradrenergic neurotransmitter functioning may be of particular significance in the context of autonomic deficits in antisocial individuals outlined earlier. Reduction of Noradrenergic functioning caused by smoking would be expected to disrupt sympathetic nervous system activity, consistent with evidence outlined earlier for reduced sympathetic arousal in antisocial individuals."

Anderson and Hoshino (2005), note that in relation to stress response systems in autism one study showed reduced Noradrenaline in urine and another study showed increased levels. They conclude that in "some autistic individuals the sympathetic nervous system may be hyper-responsive to stress" .These variable findings might be due to different subtypes not yet identified.

SEROTONIN

Beitman, Nair, and Viamontes note that Serotonin (normally) is an inhibitory brain neurochemical. Many studies have shown reduced Serotonergic function in psychopathy and in impulsivity/aggression.

Minzenberg and Siever (2006) suggest that "Serotonergic deficits are more fundamentally linked to the impulsive-antisocial features of psychopathy, but that such deficits may exert effects in the affective – interpersonal domain of psychopathy via interactions with Dopamine". This could be critical in Criminal Autistic Psychopathy.

Serotonin "inhibits the activity of amygdala projection cells" (Le Doux, 2002) and there is a tendency for low Serotonin in Antisocial Personality Disorder. Serotonin would appear to modulate or calm brain excitability and we might speculate that low Serotonin in a person with psychopathy may leave them with a more excitable brain.

In some persons with ASD Serotonin levels are high but this may not be so with Asperger's syndrome Autistic Psychopathy subtype. Millon et al (2000) note that Siever and Trestman (1993) "argue that Serotonin abnormalities are associated not only with increased aggressiveness but also with impulsiveness and inability to learn from punishment".

Although these authors link such characteristics to antisocial personality, their thesis would seem to be applicable to the sadistic personality, as well, perhaps to the explosive psychopath".

Harmer and colleagues (2003) have shown that recognition of facial expressions of fear can be specifically increased with Tryptophan or a selective Serotonin reuptake inhibitor administration, decreased with Tryptophan depletion and normalised in remitted depressed subjects with SSRIs. These findings indicate a role for Serotonergic activity in the recognition of fearful facial expressions, and neurocognitive function that is necessary for the development of moral behaviour in children, and which is impaired in children and adults with psychopathic features".

According to Bassarath (2001) "SPECT has also been used to look at the Serotonin neurotransmitter system with respect to violence". One such study found that Serotonin transporter binding in offenders was lower in the brain (Tiihonen et al, 1997). .

There is a conflict in that low Serotonin is associated with aggression and high Serotonin can be seen in autism. The Serotonin reuptake inhibitor increases Serotonin levels.

In terms of Serotonin (5 hydroxytryptamine) many studies have shown increased blood (platelet) Serotonin in autism. Nevertheless this only occurs in about 50%, which again brings up the issue of subtyping. It is possible that these are not those with Criminal Autistic Psychopathy. Nevertheless there is a great amount of work to be done on neurochemistry and sub typing will help to focus this research.

Whether the subcategory of Autistic Psychopathy subtype would show low Serotonin has not been assessed. What we have had from studies in the past have been mean levels of Serotonin. Fluoxetine, a Serotonin reuptake inhibitor, has been shown to be useful with impulsivity and autism. The Fenfluramine challenge is a marker of Serotonergic activity. O'Keane et al (1992) showed a blunted prolactin response in males with psychopathy. This blunted prolactin response links to impulsivity and not to interpersonal relating. Sonderstrom (2003) has shown that psychopathy was associated with an increased HVA/5HIAA ratio indicating deficient regulation of Dopaminergic activity".

Sonderstrom (2005) hypothesised that Serotonin modulates as well as inhibiting – "catecholaminergically driven aggression and its activity, measured by the metabolite 5HIAA in the CSF" and this shows a decrease in destructive violence.

Morrison *et al* (2004) stated that "an excessive amount of Serotonin may well cause a person to lash out with destructive behaviour" It is interesting that a proportion of persons with Autistic Psychopathy have high Serotonin . The Serotonin findings are contradictory. One might hypothesise that too little or too much Serotonin causes problems.

Toal (2005) points out that in autism there may be regional differences "in neural development (programmed cell death) may underpin a proportion of the symptoms typical of the disorder". Toal states that "the potential role of 5HT in ASD is of importance, because 5HT acts as a trophic or differentiation factor during brain development, and helps modulate social and repetitive behaviours". There are problems in Criminal Autistic Psychopathy.

Blum (1997) points out that women in general are about 30% higher in Serotonin than men, reinforcing the notion that females are less reliant on a fight response.

Pickett *et al* (2005) also note that in Asperger's syndrome "a significant reduction in cortical 5HT2a receptor binding. Reduced receptor binding has been associated with abnormal social communication."

CORTISOL

Research indicates that:

> "low resting cortisol levels to impaired fear reactivity in young children, elevated sensation seeking in adults and persistent aggressive behaviour across child and adult samples. Low cortisol does not appear to be a general correlate of antisocial behaviour or conduct disorder. Rather, it seems to be a unique feature of a small subgroup exhibiting the most persistent and severe conduct disorder presentation" (Looney *et al*, 2006).

Looney et al (2006) conclude that "males callous unemotional traits were uniquely associated with low resting cortisol levels regardless of the level of conduct problems. Furthermore, testosterone was not related to group status, supporting the discriminant validity of the cortisol-CU trait relation". This is associated with reduced sensitivity to other people's feelings.

Studies need to be carried out on cortisol in Criminal Autistic Psychopathy. In autism generally studies have shown normal or elevated levels in autism.

The relations between salivary cortisol, callous-unemotional traits and conduct problems were studied in an adolescent non-referred sample (Looney et al (2006). "In terms of gender, research currently suggests that male and female psychopathic traits are similarly associated with severe and persistent forms of aggression". Some research shows a link between callous unemotional traits and low trait anxiety.

> "Little is known about the underlying cognitive, emotional and biological correlates of female psychopathy. While the current study suggests that female CU traits (in contrast to male CU traits) may not be associated with cortisol abnormalities, caution should be taken in

providing more definitive statements and interpretation given the preliminary nature of the findings, small sample size."

"If confirmed in future investigations, it is important to note that an absence of a statistically significant CU-low cortisol relation for female participants would not entirely rule out an emotional under-reactivity component to female psychopathy."

"Male psychopathy is simply more robustly tied to low emotional reactivity (i.e. across a number of indices such as passive avoidance impairment, heart rate, hormone, and skin conductance findings)".

TESTOSTERONE

Studies have shown that in the criminal personality disorder group there are higher testosterone levels. Dolan ((1993) also points out that studies "indicate that subgroups of offenders who are characterised by violence or aggression have higher plasma testosterone than non-aggressive offenders"

Baron-Cohen *et al* (2005) point out that "if autism is an extreme of the male brain, is this the result of elevated Foetal Testosterone (FT), abnormalities in Androgen Receptor (AR) (androgens include testosterone) or the genes controlling FT, or sexually dimorphic gene expression unrelated to FT? Currently, there are six clues that FT may play a role in autism. According to Baron-Cohen et al (2005):

(1) "FT is associated with low ratios of second-to-forth digit length and a low digit length ratio is in turn associated with autism spectrum conditions".
(2) Girls with CAH manifest more autism-like traits than their unaffected sisters and show masculine tomboy behaviour.
(3) Within normal development FT is inversely correlated with behaviours that, in the extreme, would count as diagnostic symptoms of autism. These are eye contact, vocabulary development, social functioning, and narrow interests.
(4) There is preliminary evidence of somatic hyper-masculinization in autism, although a comprehensive study is needed.
(5) There is precocious puberty in boys with autism.
(6) Serotonin levels can be elevated and brain-derived neurotrophic factors (BDNF) can be elevated these are mediated by FT."

In my view it may be that the ultimate male brain is the Criminal Autistic Psychopathy.

According to Warren *et al* Langevin (1991 there was "a trend towards elevated level of testosterone" in sex killers.

OXYTOCIN AND VASOPRESSIN

The hormone vasopressin and oxytocin are involved in attachment behaviour. If this hormone oxytocin is blocked in certain animals "she mates but does not bond" (Le Doux,

2002). This is not unlike what the human sexual predator does although the transfer of this animal hormonal information to humans needs further study. Male bonding is associated with vasopressin and female bonding with oxytocin.

According to Tancredi (2005):

> "there are basic differences in their reward circuitries of lust and social bonding, the neurohormones involved in both these emotional conditions affect each other. Increases in testosterone, which is important for sex drive, lust, and sexual pleasure, can under certain conditions increase both vasopressin and oxytocin levels, thus ensuring that sexual pleasure enriches the possibility of attachment. Conversely, increases in oxytocin and vasopressin can result in greater amounts of circulating testosterone, ensuring that attachment can bring about lust. When this happens, feelings of attachment and romance will trigger sexual desires".

Normal attachment and romance does not feature in serial killing.

Some have speculated that testosterone enhances the growth of the right hemisphere, thus increasing the size of this hemisphere, whereas in females the left hemisphere is larger. The specialisation of the two hemispheres – the right involved with the systematising and spatial ability, and the left with empathy and language – creates a laterality affect, a differential of abilities between the two sides, which explains the cluster of abilities that are predominantly found in the male brain and those in the female brain" (Tancredi, 2005)

Hines (2004) points out that in relation to androgen what does appear to be associated with testosterone is antisocial, delinquent, of problem behaviours, such as substance abuse, job and relationship problems, military absence without leave, stealing, and divorce". She states that:

> "the internal cognitive state most associated with aggression is the presence of hostile thoughts. The internal affective states associated with aggression include, in particular hostile and angry feelings. Thus, at this level, similar to the level of person and situation, hormones-induced predispositions to experience hostile feelings and thoughts could increase aggressive behaviour."

She hypothesises that:

> "including the possibility that androgen exposure leads to increased perceptions, expectations, or attributions of hostility, to increase narcissism, to increase arousal, or to increased engagement in activities that promote hostile or aggressive thoughts and feelings."

She controversially states that "the more likely that aggression, or factors associated with it, influence levels of testosterone than that testosterone influences aggression in adulthood" It is possible that internal and external factors are operating in relation to testosterone.

The neurochemicals involved with these circuits affect one another. An increase in testosterone and Dopamine, which is important for sexual drive, can result in an increase in vasopressin and oxytocin, increases in these neurochemicals responsible for social bonding can result in greater circulating levels of the neurochemicals of lust. However, if the neurochemicals of lust reach excessive levels, they will dampen the circulating levels of the neurochemicals of social bonding. The converse is also true. Therefore, some individuals with elevated levels of testosterone or Dopamine will be unable to experience to social bonding.

They will seek out sexual contact, but never allow attachment to occur. Hormones and their influence on the brain may render the individual incapable of controlling sexual impulses. Serial killers have problems with perverse sadistic sexual impulses.

LUTENIZING HORMONE

Moir and Jessel (1995) describe:

> "the hormonal profiles of some 49 cases of extreme sexual aggression were studied, and surprising high levels of lutenizing hormone – a pattern that is more feminine than masculine – were discovered."

There is evidence that in women the hippocampus and frontal cortex are larger, that there are more neurons in the temporal cortex dealing with language.

EVOLUTIONARY PSYCHOLOGY AND SERIAL KILLERS

In the wider world diversity is seen as important. In our world the serial killers can only have a negative position. Whether there could be other environments where they could prosper or thrive different from ours and where their behaviour would be evolutionary adaptive is a difficult question. It is probably useful behind enemy lines in war.

According to Sullivan et al (2006), the trickster:

> "possesses no values, moral or social, is at the mercy of his passions and appetite . . he inflicts great damage on those around him and also suffers innumerable blows, defeats, indignities, and dangers resulting from his thoughtless, reckless forays"

The Yorubas in Nigeria have a word for psychopath called Arankan. Murphy describes this person as someone who "always goes his own way regardless of others, who is uncooperative, full of malice, and bull headed". Murphy (1976) also describes psychopathy in the Alaskan Inuit Eskimos as kunlangeta who has:

> "a mind knows what to do but he does not do it . . it might be applied to a man who, for example, repeatedly lies and cheats and steals things and does not go hunting and, when the other men are out of the village, takes sexual advantage of many women, someone who does not pay attention to reprimands and who is always being brought to the elders for punishment."

The Alaskan form of execution is to push the man into the water from the ice on hunting expeditions.

Criminal Autistic Psychopathy can have probably a value if a society is in great turmoil, if it is in a war like situation, if it is under attack from predators where the fearless Autistic Psychopathy is probably better at defending the group than the more balanced individual. In Criminal Autistic Psychopathy is self-defeating and self-damaging in peacetime and in peacetime is not evolutionary adaptive except in very small doses. In very mild Autistic Psychopathy probably gives an edge probably in business and politics where fearlessness, a certain lack of empathy, a certain daring, and a certain capacity to take risks can be highly advantageous. It is probably because of this that these genes have therefore been selected out and are continuing. Some of these people as well have been greater discoverers and of course societies who have a capacity to develop weapons of warfare tend to be more successful in the competitive world. World history is a history of groups fighting each other, it is a competitive world. The world from a historical point of view has been survival of the fittest.

If there is a shortage of food the psychopath kills other members and therefore survives. It therefore leads to primitive survival.

Chapter 10

SERIAL KILLERS

DEFINITION AND DESCRIPTION

Thomas Hobbes (1651) wrote of the course of human life as being "solitary, poor, nasty, brutish, and short". An early description of a serial killer comes from the Bible Psalms 10: 7 – 9:

> "His mouth is full of curses and lies and threats: trouble and evil are under his tongue. He lies in wait near the villages; from ambush he murders the innocent, watching in secret for his victims He lies in wait like a lion in cover; he lies in wait to catch the helpless; he catches the helpless and drags them off in his net. His victims are crushed, they collapse: they fall under his strength."

The definition of serial murder varies from those who committed more than one murder to those who have committed more than ten. The duration between murders is also a subject of controversy, which goes from hours to days. Ressler *et al* (1993) define serial murder as:

> "three or more separate events with an emotional cooling off period between homicides, each murder taking place at a different location."

According to Cawthorne (2002), for the FBI to be described as a serial killer one has to have killed four people over a period. A spree killer is somebody that goes into a restaurant and shoots a lot of people.

Kelleher *et al* (1998) define serial murder as:

> "The act of murdering three or more individuals in a period of 30 days or more."

There can be and often are quiescent periods between killing. They note that a broader definition of serial killing would be "the murder of at least three individuals in which each lethal act was separated from the next by a discrete cooling off period". (Kelleher & Kelleher, 1998)

There is a difference between multiple murderers that often includes women and sadistic serial killers who mutilate and torture the bodies. The sadistic serial killers are more likely to have Criminal Autistic Psychopathy.

According to Ressler *et al* (1993) sexual homicide is a homicide that was "sexual in nature" and involved involvement with sexual aspects of the body. Sexual murder involves anger, sadism, and lust. They noted that the "sadistic murderer kills as part of ritualised, sadistic fantasies". There is a dangerous fusion of sexuality and aggression in the sadistic serial murderer.

Warren *et al* (1996) point out that "the serial killer has to demonstrate an enduring pattern of sexual arousal to images of suffering or humiliation, and (b) the offender killed at least three victims in at least three incidents separated by time, place or both".

Moir *et al* (1995) describe a sadistic sex murderer as someone who is probably under 35, introverted a loner, close attachment to his mother and "a bad relationship with his distant father". This profile is close enough to Criminal Autistic Psychopathy.

PREVALENCE SERIAL KILLER

There are widely varying estimates of the prevalence of serial killing. According to Simon (1996), the "FBI estimates that there are 500 serial killers at large who kill at least 3,500 people each year. Another more conservative estimate has the death toll from 200 serial killers at 2,000 people at each year – approximately 10% of all murders" The serial killers are sometimes seen as recreational killers. Simon describes women who kill serially as "serial enterprise killers" and that less than 5% of serial killers are women. The general age range is twenties to mid thirties.

Depue (2005) stated that "Serial killers are a miniscule percentage of the population, maybe 30 of them wandering the US at any one time, out of more than 250 million people".

Morrison and Goldberg (2004) estimated that there were 35 serial killers in the United States at any one time. They pointed out that in terms of motivationless murders that "between 1976 and 1984 there was a 160% increase in murders with unknown motives". According to Prentky (1989), certainly copycat phenomenon will always play a role.

From media reports, Harbort and Mokros (2001) estimated that between 1990 and 1995 there were worldwide "212 serial murders that had killed 2,400 victims". It has possibly increased in frequency recently.

Leyton (1989) describes two multiple murderers occurring in the 1920s rising to over 20 in the 1980s. Clearly these are only very approximate figures. Multiple murdering is different from serial killing in that it mostly lacks the sadistic component.

SOCIAL PROFILE OF SERIAL KILLERS

Warren *et al* (1996) stated that

> "65% of the sample came from middle, or upper middleclass families". The characteristics of 20 sexually sadistic serial murderers included 55% having homosexual experience in adulthood, 45% showing a paraphiliac interest in peeping, obscene phone calls and indecent exposure, 25% being interested in fetishism, bondage, and transvestism, 80% showing evidence of violent fantasies, and 75% showing violent theme collections."

They did not find a higher rates amongst blacks.

Warren *et al* (1996) point out that "85% of the sample had violent fantasies that seemed to remain consistent over significant periods of time. These fantasies contain a ritualised, repetitious core that is highly arousing to the sexual sadist". Hazelwood *et al (1993)* pointed out that "sexual sadists are particularly adept at seducing women into becoming compliant accessories to their violent fantasies or criminal acts."

FACTORS ASSOCIATED WITH SERIAL KILLING

Harbort and Mokros (1986) found that "serial murders have a higher likelihood of personality disorder, cerebral anomalies, and offence premeditation and are more likely to have had no relationship with the victim prior to the offence" as compared to single murders. This situation is even more pronounced in serial sex murders.

Leyton (1986) stated "that serial killers are interested in both "revenge and a life-long celebrity career" in a social context that highlights worldly ambition, success and failure, and "manly avenging violence". This is in addition to the thrill seeking.

Schizophrenia is extremely rare in serial killers but they are often misdiagnosed as being psychotic. People can't imagine a non-psychotic person engaging in serial killing. They often keep a souvenirs items of clothing or body parts of the person they kill. To the outside world they can present a normal façade or false selves. They are persons with multiple selves or identity diffusion.

According to Haire (1952), in relation to sexual murder he notes that "butchers and hunters are frequently represented in the list of murderers. In the course of their profession they lose the aversion to killing that the normal human being experiences, and in the act of killing animals they discover, in most cases by accident and to their own surprise – the usual feature in the acquirement of sexual perversions – that killing gives them pleasure, and this arouses in them the desire to murder" .

De River (1956) is largely wrong about the juvenile sadist and for his belief that parental rearing factors are critical between four and five years of age. In the case of the serial killer of course the genetic factors are critical. And in the case of the serial criminal psychopathic killer parental factors in terms of interpersonal factors play a very small role. Of course parental genes are of massive importance here. Environmental factors play a secondary role.

Serial killers can be very interested in police work and particularly with the power and control police officers have. Some have even joined the police for a period.

FANTASY AND SERIAL KILLING

Goya wrote that "fantasy abandoned by reason produces impossible monsters . . united with her, she is the mother of the arts and the origin of their marvels". (Storr, 1992).

Serial killers are often "Walter Mitty" types. MacCulloch *et al* (1983) emphasised the issue of control and "the repeated practice of behaviour and fantasy which is characterised by a wish to control another person by domination, denigration, or inflicting pain for the purpose of producing mental pleasure and sexual arousal in the sadist".

MacCulloch *et al* (1983) showed that:

> "81% of the offenders had been masturbating to fantasies of rape, buggery, kidnap, bondage, flagellation, torture, and killing for extended periods of time before their offences. The majority of the offenders reported non-aggressive sexual fantasies following puberty, but one to seven years after the onset of puberty, sadistic content began to appear, accompanied by a substantial increase in masturbatory activity. Significant number of the offenders described their sadistic fantasies as being progressive in nature with the fantasies continually being changed to maintain their efficacy as a source of arousal and pleasure."

They also noted that the "increase in the power of fantasies was accompanied by increasing the sadistic context and also by including fantasy based on previous behavioural 'tryouts' of the main fantasy sequence" They also point out that "fantasy of successful control and dominance of the world can be conceptualised as an operant which increases the probability of its own recurrence by the relief which it gives from a pervasive sense of failure" They also elaborate that: "if a man presents with sadistic sexual fantasies, admits previous tryouts, and demonstrates a pattern of progression of offending and fantasy, then progression to killing would appear to be a strong possibility".

Grubin (1997) also notes that the FBI "demonstrated that fantasy was indeed an important driving force in the motivation behind the offending of a group of serious, serial offenders". Grubin points out that "fantasy may be a sensitive indicator of risk, but it is unclear how specific it is". This is a reasonable point. Prentky *et al* (1983) believe that fantasy as an internal drive mechanism for repetitive acts of sexual violence and hypothesised "that an intrusive fantasy life manifested in higher prevalence of paraphilias, documented or self-reported violent fantasies, and organised crime scenes in the serial murderers".

Abel and Blanchard (1974) were in agreement that there was a "high concordance between the presence of deviant fantasies and the occurrence of deviant behaviour".

The Burgess model, as described by Prentky et *al* (1983), of sexual homicide fits in well with Criminal Autistic Psychopathy. This model has "impaired development of attachments in early life; patterned responses that serve to generate fantasies; a private, internal world that is consumed with violent thoughts and leaves the person isolated and self preoccupied; and a feedback filter that sustains repetitive thinking patterns"(Prentky *et al*, 1983).

Prentky *et al* (1983) showed that the internal drive mechanism showed "a higher prevalence of paraphilias, a higher prevalence of organised crime scenes, and a higher prevalence of violent fantasies". They showed that "violent fantasy was present in 86% of multiple (or serial) murderers and only 23% of single murderers". They point out that "the more the fantasy is rehearsed, the more power it acquires and the stronger the association between the fantasy content and sexual arousal". They also point out that there is some evidence that fetishism and transvestism are more often associated with sexual aggression than other paraphilias. Fetishists are also more into sadomasochism.

Langevin *et al* (1985) pointed out that sadomasochistic fantasies in conjunction with a high degree of force might be premonitory signs of extreme dangerousness including sexual murder. They conclude that "of all those who harbour sadistic fantasies, only a small (unknown) fraction attempt to play out their fantasies. The presence of fantasy alone is a relatively poor harbinger of future conduct" Fantasy plays a much smaller role in the disorganised offender as compared to the organised offender.

IDENTITY DIFFUSION AND SERIAL KILLER

Serial killers tend to be Jekyll and Hyde figures. They have multiple selves but no coherent sense of self. According to Moir and Jessel (1995), "representing the nightmare extreme of masculine violence, it is intriguing to find that researchers have identified a definite trace of the feminine in a significant proportion of such killers" There is often sexual identity diffusion. They are very narcissistic and male and female identities can be somewhat diffuse in them although they are obviously primarily male.

PERVERSION AND SERIAL KILLING

According to Haire (1952), "originally the word perversion was useful. It is derived from a Latin word which means turn the side, and denotes a sexual desire or a sexual activity which diverges from the most usual one". "The vast majority of persons, at some time or other, indulge in sexual outlets which are commonly described as abnormal or perverse, though their most frequent outlet is usually described as normal"

In discussing sadism, De River (1951) states that algolagnia "has the correlative impulsive, masochism, derives its name from von Sacher-Masoch. A more appropriate name has been suggested by Eulenburg, a term which was coined by von Schrenck-Notzing, who used the name algolagnia, algos meaning pain, and lagneia meaning lust".

De River also discusses lust murder as showing that:

> "Death has occurred through torture, with the characteristic marks of the degenerate killer, i.e. mutilation of the genitals, biting, dissection, the amputation of the parts, slashing of the abdomen, with exposure of abdominal viscera and many times evisceration. Frequently the killer, in a wild state of frenzy, will slash and mutilate the intestines, often removing by incision or pulling out the intestines. However, we find little difference between lust, murder and sadistic homicide, other than the fact that in lust murder there is mutilation of the genitals, and that sadistic homicide is but the expression of a comparatively milder form of criminal sadism"

> "The true lust murderer remains in the heat of passion, and the crime as in sadistic homicide, is usually premeditated. The crime of murder in these cases is brought about to relieve sexual tension and the lust murderer only gains satisfaction through the physical injury or torture of the victim."

Serial killers can show evidence of exhibitionism or voyeurism, transvestism or fetishism. They find the degradation of human beings incredibly exciting. They hate and are bored by respectful human interaction. They are contemptuous of values like respect, care, tolerance, and all positive human values. They can show autistic charms with women, which is surprising but true.

Tancredi (2005) points out that "what lust is combined with anger it can result in violent acts – rape, assault and even murder"

Krafft-Ebing (1965) discusses hyperaesthesia (abnormally increased sexual desire). He points out that the:

"commission of these atrocious acts by degenerated and partially defective individuals is the outcome of an irresistible impulse or delirium. The mechanism of these actions is indeed the property of psychical degeneration."

It was an error to talk of degeneration but Krafft-Ebing was writing in the 19th century.

The driven compulsive impulse of the serial killer as described by Krafft-Ebing (1965) is also described in St. Paul's letter to the Romans, Book V:

"what I do is not what I want to do . . it is no longer I who perform the action, but sin that lodges in me. For I know that nothing good lodges in me . . what I do is against my will . . clearly it is no longer I who am the agent, but sin that has its lodging in me."

Krafft-Ebing (1965) discusses the paraesthesia of sexual feeling (perversion of the sexual instinct).

"In this condition there is perverse emotional colouring of the sexual ideas. Ideas physiologically and psychologically accompanied by feelings of disgust, give rise to pleasurable sexual feelings; and the abnormal association finds expression in passionate, uncontrollable emotions. The practical results are perverse acts (perversion of the sexual instinct)."

Krafft-Ebing (1965) further points out that:

"sadism is the experience of sexual pleasurable sensations (including orgasm) produced by acts of cruelty, bodily punishment, afflicted in one owns person or when witnessed in others, be they animals or human beings. It may also consist of an innate desire to humiliate, hurt, wound or even destroy others in order thereby to create sexual pleasure in ones self."

Harbort and Mokros (2001) point out in their study from Germany that: "some authors have equated serial murderers with sex killers or lust murderers" . There was a great deal of mutilation of various parts of the body particularly the sexual organs. Nevertheless in this German sample, only one third of the samples were sexual murderers. Clearly not all serial murderers have a sexual motive. The serial killers tended to be younger. Neither did many of them have clear single modus operandi. A quarter of these sexual murderers used strangulation, another quarter bludgeoning, and a quarter stabbing. They had multiple sexual perversions by and large. Just under half showed a number of sexual deviations. Over 30% showed sadism and another 30% showed fetishism. Clearly some murderers were attracted only to persons of one gender or one age group. In America, Bundy, the serial killer who will be described later, was interested in girls who parted their hair in the middle of their forehead. In Europe 13% of the serial sexual murderers showed some anatomical preference.

SERIAL KILLERS AND SOCIAL RELATIONSHIPS

In their earlier life, serial killers are not uncommonly sadistic, perverse and cruel to siblings and other children. They are not uncommonly cruel and can kill animals before they start killing humans.

Hazelwood *et al* (1993) pointed out that "sexual sadists are particularly adept at seducing women into becoming compliant accessories to their violent fantasies or criminal acts". They have psychopathic or autistic charm.

In *Clinical Psychiatry* written by Mayer-Gross, Slater, and Roth (1960), they wrote that:

> "the social legal importance of the emotionally callous psychopath is considerable . . . this quality of personality contributes to the makeup of societies most ruthless, dangerous and incorrigible criminals. However it must not be assumed that the emotionally callous are invariably criminal . . . their lack of capacity for human feeling and their lack of need for the affection, the friendship and the understanding of others, is like a blind spot of personality" They also point out that the callous psychopath will have been found to be "generally unresponsive, incapable of friendship, or even of a natural affection to his parents. For reasons, into which genetic and environmental causes may both enter, his parents have frequently shown some of the same traits too."

Many of those features would fit with Autistic Psychopathy, Criminal Autistic Psychopathy, and General Psychopathy.

The kind of persons we are discussing here tend to be loners and to be shy with huge empathy deficits in interpersonal relationships. They are immature personalities and have major problems in reciprocal social relationships. They are contemptuous of people and relate to them on a part-object relationship, which means they dehumanise people. People are there to be used. Nevertheless they are very sensitive to human rejection, which can lead to a fall in their self-esteem and an episode of serial killing to boost self-esteem. They are good at recognising defenceless vulnerable victims for their killing pleasure. For different serial killers pleasure can come from different aspects of the process. They are callous and unemotional in relation to people and have been that way since childhood.

Woodworth and Porter (2002) describe one psychopathic offender who "had decided to murder an ex-girlfriend because he felt she was interfering with his new relationship, and he simply decided that murdering her would help resolve this issue" This is the kind of strategy that a person with Criminal Autistic Psychopathy would engage in. It shows seriously defective problem solving skills.

According to Haslam and Reichter (2005), serial killers with Criminal Autistic Psychopathy are not subject to the "prosocial and enriching aspects of groups" They are not capable of this form of social learning. The lack of eye contact probably increases this but is far more fundamental than that. Serial killers don't engage with the shared values of the world. They are not interested in "collective self-realisation".

Grubin showed that with murderers "about half were loners who were not part of a peer group, and that as adults about a third were literally socially isolated with little if any interaction with other people. About half were living alone at the time of their offences" This would fit with Criminal Autistic Psychopathy. Boss (1949), in a discussion of sexual perversions noted that they had a "wall of grey class" separating them from the external world.

They can be close to mother or indeed mother's boys. They can make relationships in prisons with people like themselves. Their problems with mentalisation and poor reflective function mean that they have huge problems seeing other people as human beings. They feel most alive during a killing or shortly afterwards. They fear close interpersonal relationships and are hypersensitive to criticism, somewhat paranoid of people, and blame others for their misfortunes. They are self-obsessed narcissistic and egocentric.

Meloy and Gacono (1998) note that in sexual homicide perpetrators "attachment was abnormal and mostly absent . . . [and] about one third of the sexual homicide perpetrators were abnormally hungry for attachment" In my view killing and eating their victims is a form of abnormal attachment behaviour and social hunger or neediness and wish for control. It is a way of merging with their victims. Abnormal attachment behaviour is a feature of Criminal Autistic Psychopathy and is caused particularly in Type 1 Psychopathy (Primary) by the condition.

THE KILLING PROCESS

Years before a killing takes place they may have sadistic fantasies that then progress to fantasies of killing and then later actual killing. They are and become driven to kill and addicted to the "buzz" of killing. The period between killings shortens as they get older because the "buzz" of killing lasts a shorter period and they get careless about their modus operandi. Before a killing they spend a period hunting for a suitable victim, use want ads etc.

They can also be involved in parallel in non-homicidal criminal behaviour. The killing episode may have been triggered by rejection by a woman or some other rejection. When they get a victim they generally like to kill slowly. They are organised and often have a regular modus operandi. Guns generally are not used because this killing is too quick and too impersonal. Slow strangulation is a favourite as it allows a prolonged experience of death. Multiple stabbings or beatings are also not uncommon. Penetrations of the vagina or anus may also be part of the process. For some the major excitement is the killing. For others it is the mutilation and abuse of the corpse after killing with further sexual activity or indeed cutting up the corpse and sometimes eating it. Taking photographs at all stages is not uncommon as it allows the perpetrator to relive the experience later and to masturbate to the photographs. Audiotape recordings have also been taken to record the whole process.

In terms of the acts that the serial killers commit Warren *et al* (1996) point out that 95% showed careful planning of offences, 15% showed impersonation of a police officer, 80% use a con or ruse approaching a victim, 65% kept their victims in captivity for 24 hours or more, 100% of the victims were blindfolded or gagged, 95% there was sexual bondage of the victim, 65% anal intercourse, 65% foreign object penetration, 90% a variety of sexual acts, 95% penile penetration, stabbing as a primary method of killing was in 30% and asphyxiation, and taking things belonged to victims occurred in 65%, and partner assistant crime occurred in 20%.

Warren *et al* (1996) point out that one of the people they studied who had killed stated:

> "I stood there looking at him on the ground and I suddenly had feelings of power. I realised I held this man's life in my hands . . I thought "I am like god . . I too have the power to give life or take it away" . . . I got down on my knees and took the rock and hit him again as hard as I could I watched his forehead cave in from the force of the blow and the blood and brains splattered all over the road . . I never thought it would be so easy to kill a person, or that I would enjoy it. But it was easy and I was enjoying the feeling of supremacy. A supremacy like I had never known before."

Warren *et al* (1996) state that another man who murdered "by manual strangulation told of breathing air into his dying victim so that he could watch more closely the dawning realisation that he was, in fact, going to kill her".

When caught they sometimes want to be famous, to be the greatest killers and have media coverage. Bailey (1997) notes that Krafft-Ebing suggested that "mastering and possessing an absolutely defenceless human object is the key element in sadism". Here Krafft-Ebing was describing the 19th century criminal autistic psychopathic killers. He emphasised the importance of control and dominance. This is central to Criminal Autistic Psychopathy. This includes humiliating and degrading the victims as well as the sexual excitement caused by the above. The moment the victim expired can be a peak sexual experience for these people. The killing is then a form of self-esteem regulation for them. Later they will often revisit the scene of the killing or the graves of their victims particularly on the anniversary of the killing. When eventually caught they will often reliably confess to many killings and often show very good memories of these facts.

De River (1956) describes a sadistic paedophile who ate "a fairly good dinner and had a very good nights sleep" after killing. This particular man "expressed a thrill when he saw his victims die, and admitted that the sight and odour of blood of young females has satisfied his lustful nature" He showed shallow affect. He was fascinated by newspaper accounts of his crime. He confessed totally. He was executed. He brutally killed three little girls.

NECROPHILIA

Necrophilia is a sexual interest in corpses. Wulffen (1910) described lust murder or necrosadism "in which murder precedes the sexual act with the corpse, necrostuprum in which the corpse is stolen, and necrophagy in which the corpse is mutilated and parts of it eaten". Sexual interference with bodies tends to be more common among "mortuary attendants, hospital orderlies, and grave diggers".

Herodotus noted that "It appears that sexual interference with the dead was known and abhorred by the "Egyptians". (De Slincourt, 1992)

According to De Slincourt (1992):

"When the wife of a distinguished man dies, or any woman who happens to be beautiful or well known, her body is not given to the embalmers immediately, but only after the lapse of three or four days. This is a precautionary measure prevent the embalmers from violating her corpse, a thing this is actively said to have happened."

According to Stephen Hucker (1990), in William Faulkner's Story: *A Rose for Emily* "a woman keeps the corpse of her former lover lying in her bed at home". This may be related to a grief reaction. Krafft-Ebing (1965) noted that "there is undoubtedly direct preference for a corpse to a living woman".

Hirschfeld (1952) stated that a person who kills and then sexually abuses the body shows a "frenzied intensification of the aggressive and destructive impulse. The murderer is not satisfied by merely killing his victim; he also wants to possess her and destroy her beyond death".

Hucker (1990) points out that:

"Paraphilias are characterised by arousal in response to sexual objects or situations that are not part of normative arousal – activity patterns and whose essential features are intense sexual urges and sexually arousing fantasies generally involving non-human objects, the suffering or humiliation of one's self or one's partner, or children or other non-consenting persons."

Gerontophilia is the sexual "preference for older partners". Rossman and Resnick (1989) point out that "necrophilia was considered by the Catholic Church to be neither whoring (fornicatio) nor bestiality, but pollution with a tendency to whoring". They also note that: "Cannibalistic tribal rituals are based on the notion that consumption of human flesh parts imparts a special power of strength to the cannibal". They also point out "that King Herod had sex with his wife Marianne for seven years after he killed her" (this is a legend). The genuine necrophile has a persistent sexual attraction to corpses. They describe necrophilic homicide as murder "to obtain a corpse for sexual purposes" Regular necrophilia is the use of an already dead body for sexual pleasure and necrophilic fantasy is the fantasying about sexual activity with corpses.

Bartholomew *et al* (1978) state that the total control over the corpse is often seen as important. Others see the lack of rejection by the corpse as important. Some necrophiliacs engage in this because they are frightened of rejection, others do it because they want company, others do it for the power. Bartholomew *et al* (1978) describe the case of a man who eventually completed suicide who was a "very retiring, shy lad, who exhibited a number of nervous symptoms, a stammer, and a facial tic being the most obvious" He was described as being a schizoid type and was depressed. He killed a boy and had anal intercourse following death. There was a view expressed that one couldn't engage in this without being psychotic at the time. This is not true. Browne (1875) stated that in relation to necrophilia "such aberrations owe their origin to that state of privation, degradation, or degeneration, as the case may be, from which all races have sprung, and to which, were the inhibitive influence of religion, education, and civilisation withdrawn, all races would inevitably return".

Diagnoses that have been given to necrophiliacs include schizophrenia and personality disorders. Rossman and Resnick's (1989) sample of necrophiliacs found that "the rate of homicide committed by true necrophiles was 28%" Prostitutes are sometimes paid to pretend they are dead.

There are probably higher rates in people who have contact with corpses like embalmers. They are mostly male. It can occur at all IQ levels. Rossman and Resnick (1989) note that about half have "unusual beliefs - Para religious beliefs or devil worship.

"The most common motive of the true necrophile was to possess an unresisting and unrejecting partner. Other commonly reported motives were: reunion with a romantic partner; conscious sexual attraction to corpses; attempt to gain comfort and to overcome feelings of isolation; attempt to gain self-esteem by the expression of power over a homicide victim. Less commonly reported motives were: unavailability of a living partner; compensation for a fear of women; belief that sex with a living woman was a mortal sin; need to achieve feelings of total control over a sexual partner."

About half engaged in vaginal intercourse; 11% in anal intercourse; 11% in fallacio or cunnilingus; 30% in mutilation; and 6% in necrophagia.

Chapter 11

FEMALE SERIAL KILLERS ARE RARE

According to Jones (2002), Kipling is reported to have said that "the female of the species" being "deadlier than the male". Female serial killers do exist even though they are much rarer than males. Female Criminal Autistic Psychopathy does exist. Nevertheless Simon (1996) states, "I am not aware of the existence of any true female serial sexual killers". There is little doubt that killing can serve multiple functions for an individual and does exist in families.

Daly and Wilson (1988) found that male to male homicide was 30 to 40 times that of female on female homicide.

Kelleher and Kelleher (1998) point out that there are female serial killers:

"who are far more lethal – and often, far more successful in their determination to kill – than their male counterparts."

They describe the female serial killer as quiet "who is often painstakingly methodological and eminently lethal in her actions". They identified almost 100 female serial killers in the past 100 years. Of critical importance they point out that the female serial killer "rarely commits a sexual homicide". This is what separates them very much from the male serial killer.

Nevertheless the female serial killer shows gross lack of empathy and is extremely callous. People do not think of women as serial killers. They are therefore not identified as quickly as males. Hickey (1991) points out that female serial killers are:

"the quiet killers. They are every bit as lethal as male serial murderers, but we are seldom aware one is in the midst because of the low visibility of their killing."

Kelleher and Kelleher (1998) note that female serial killers often continue their acts for up to slightly over eight years while male serial killers kill for about four years in their acts. Only about 5% of the victims are children. In killers where there is more than one person involved tend to be a bit younger while the average age for other female serial killers is usually starting at about age 30. While the male serial killer often targets strangers the female serial killer will often target somebody whom they know.

Female serial killers often have titles like "Borgia", "beautiful", and "grandma". *Webster's New Universal Dictionary* defines a black widow as "a poisonous spider of the genus Latrodectus, especially the female, which devours its mate".

Kelleher and Kelleher (1998) define a black widow as:

> "a woman who systematically murders multiple spouses, partners, other family members, or individuals outside of the family with whom she has developed a personal relationship."

The black widow is often quite intelligent and meticulous in her planning. Poison would be by far her most common method of killing with women. The black widow can also use suffocation or strangulation. Shooting of victims would be rare by women. The killing is often for profit with women.

According to Kelleher and Kelleher (1998), the next category of female serial killers is that of angels of death who like the male variety Joseph Mengele, the Nazi doctor who had this title. He decided who would go to the work camps and decided who would die immediately at the entrance of the concentration camps. Angels of death tend to work as nurses or in the care of unwell people, or people with disability. Again poisoning would be a common method of killing for them.

Another type of female killer is the revenge type. An American who received the name the Borgia of America poisoned members of her family and extended family because she was not allowed to get married to a person of her choice.

A very controversial form of killing now is called Munchausen Syndrome by proxy. A number of mothers had been accused of killing their infants and these accusations have not been supported, and these mothers were falsely imprisoned. This phenomenon does occur, but it is rare and professionals have to be very careful to avoid making false accusations. These mothers are accused of making their infants ill and one often finds that mother is depressed or wants attention etc.

Corvin (1952) records a case from the 1840s when a London nursemaid who confessed that she had killed animals and children for no other reason than it gave her a peculiar indescribable pleasure. She derived sexual satisfaction from the sight of her victim's death agonies. She had indulged her urge to kill for years before her crimes were discovered, and had killed many victims in secret.

Wulffen (1952) is of the opinion that the typically feminine equivalent of sexual murder is poisoning. He points out that "women poisoners frequently take pleasure in their nefarious activities. Psychologically this is explicable, as the need for secrecy and methodological procedure in obtaining the poison, the preparation of the potion, and anticipation of the result involve considerable preoccupation and may therefore give satisfaction. For instance, Margaret Gottfried, who poisoned a number of people, confessed that she experienced considerable pleasure in poisoning."

DIFFERENCES IN MALE AND FEMALE BRAIN STRUCTURE

Females in general tend to be somewhat less aggressive than males. Female aggression is more subtle. The structure of the female and male brains is different and this probably plays a role in the lower levels of violence and killing in females.

GENDER DIFFERENCES IN DEVELOPMENT OF BRAIN STRUCTURE

Looney *et al.* (2006) state that:

> "In terms of gender, research currently suggests that male and female psychopathic traits are similarly associated with severe and persistent forms of aggression".

Some research shows a link between callous unemotional traits and low trait anxiety. Looney *et al.* conclude that for:

- "males callous unemotional traits were uniquely associated with low resting cortisol levels regardless of the level of conduct problems. Furthermore, testosterone was not related to group status, supporting the discriminant validity of the cortisol-CU trait relation.
- Little is known about the underlying cognitive, emotional and biological correlates of female psychopathy.
- If confirmed in future investigations, it is important to note that an absence of a statistically significant CU-low cortisol relation for female participants would not entirely rule out an emotional under-reactivity component to female psychopathy".
- Male psychopathy is simply more robustly tied to low emotional reactivity (i.e. across a number of indices such as passive avoidance impairment, heart rate, hormone, and skin conductance findings)."

While male brains are slightly heavier, they are less integrated in terms of long range interconnections of nerve cells. Women have a larger corpus callosum that is connecting nerve cells between the two sides of the brain. This improves integration in the female brain. In the male brain, cells tend to be more tightly placed. Women have better language skills than men and language tends to be a little more bilateral in female brains

Baron-Cohen *et al* (2005) note that males are better at systematising and at engineering and mechanics while females are better at empathising including being more sensitive to other people and being better at recognising emotions in other people. Females have more developed human characteristics and therefore are less likely to behave in a dehumanising killing fashion but they can do it.

Baron-Cohen *et al* (2005) state that:

> "the cerebrum as a whole is about 9% larger in men and is also larger in boys, a difference that is driven more by white matter than by grey."

Despite the larger total volume of white matter in men (and despite the conflicting studies of sex differences in specific corpus callosum measures), three-dimensional Morphometry suggests that the ratio of corpus callosum to total cerebral volume is actually smaller in men. This is consistent with the finding that increased brain size predicts a decrease inter-hemispheric connectivity and that larger brains come with proportionally smaller corpora callosal in humans and other species. Reports of anatomically localised cerebral sexual dimorphism are less consistent, but the male amygdala undergoes an extended period of growth during childhood; it is larger in boys and may remain larger in men. These anatomical differences likely result from differences in micro architecture. There are more neurons in the male cerebral cortex, and in general, these neurons are more densely packed, albeit with some regional exceptions."

They go on to point out that:

> "overall, greater numbers and denser packing of neurons, together with more intra-hemispheric white matter projecting from these neurons, indirectly suggest the pattern of increased local connectivity and decreased intra-hemispheric or (long range) connectivity in the male brain. Physiological observations, thus far, seem consistent with this picture; language-related activation in female brains is more bilateral, suggesting greater inter-hemispheric connectivity."

It is possible that some of the factors account for the low rate of female serial killers.

In Autistic Psychopathy there is increased local connectivity and reduced long-range connectivity. This is associated with a larger brain.

According to Baron-Cohen *et al* (2005), this is more associated with the extreme male brain. I believe that the factors mentioned play a role in homicide in some cases of criminal Autistic Psychopathy. Problems with the amygdala are clearly relevant and Baron-Cohen *et al* (2005) note that:

> "the development of the amygdala in autism likewise seems an extreme of typical male brain development. In children with autism between 18 and 35 months old, the amygdala is abnormally large, even when corrected for total brain volume. The enlargement persists throughout early childhood exactly during the period of sex-differential amygdala growth in normal boys. By the time children with autism reach adolescence, the enlargement has disappeared; by early adulthood the amygdala in autism is abnormally small."

Chapter 12

TREATMENT OR INCARCERATION?

Serial killers often need to be locked up for the protection of society and not as punishment as their abnormal brain functioning has undermined their ability to be sensitive to their victims. The treatment problem is their inability to learn from experience and therefore from psychological treatment. Autobiographical memory problems are part of this problem.

Depue (2005) states that:

> "Once evil has taken hold in a person, it becomes too powerful to reverse. The same was true of certain sexual predators, especially the serial sexual sadist."
>
> "Once the most basic of all human urges, the sexual urge, merges completely with violence, the link can never be broken. The damage is irreversible."

Harris and Rice (2006) point out that:

> "There is no evidence that any treatments yet applied to psychopaths have been shown to be effective in reducing violence or crime. In fact, some treatments are effective for other offenders are actually harmful for psychopaths in that they appear to promote recidivism."

Seto and Quinsey (2006) pointed out that "one matched comparison study found that psychopathic offenders are more likely to re-offend after participating in a therapeutic community programme".

Kraepelin (1968) points out that:

> "Such men are born criminals by nature, and are only distinguished from ordinary criminals by the great extent of their moral incapacity, by their having wills completely unaffected by the restraining experience of life, and by their being fundamentally incorrigible…There is therefore, as a rule, no other course to be taken, for their own sake, and for the sake of those around them, then to isolate them as being unfit for society, and as far as possible to find them occupation."

This perfectly fits the profile of a serial killer.

Nevertheless it is known that "rewiring of the brain" can occur through psychotherapeutic and pharmacological treatments. If these were implemented in childhood there is a theoretical possibility that change might be brought about. The question is whether if treatments like

Empathy Training, Mind Reading Skills Therapy, Pragmatic Language Therapy if given in an intensive programme in childhood, could they bring about significant change? I believe that this is possible. One is attempting (a massive task) to socialise the child to societal values or socializations to non-criminal values. At best one could only expect very small changes.

According to Fitzgerald (2004), there is evidence that a person with Autistic Psychopathy like Ludwig Wittgenstein did make very slow progress in the interpersonal area over his life. This is shown in the development of his philosophy, which went from a one-person philosophy in The Tractatus to a two-person philosophy in Philosophical Investigations.

Tancredi (2005) suggest futuristic treatments including introducing normal DNA into:

"The damaged cells and substituted for the abnormal form, returning the cells to normal functioning, and correcting the defect. If the DNA is so damaged that genetic therapy is too complex and not therapeutic, stem cells can effectively restore function. These cells, our new leaders are quick to add, can be introduced to replicate in the child's own body through chemical stimulation, or they can be obtained from embryo sources and inserted into damaged areas of the brain."

He also speculates that:

"Brain implants, such as neurosilicon hybrids, as well as computer chips, have been shown to substitute for injured neurons or to act at sites of stimulation of the brain. Individuals, for example, with impairment of parts of the amygdala can have that region "cured" with implants."

Raine (2002) points out that:

"Transplanted stem cells from human brains into old rats results in migration of these cells to the hippocampus, improving cognitive ability in old rats within four weeks of transplantation. It is conceivable that in the long term, adult offenders with damage to the hippocampus and prefrontal cortex might receive treatment to literally repair these brain structures, opening up the possibility of reversal of cognitive and behavioural brain deficits implicated in the aetiology of violence."

LAW AND CRIMINAL RESPONSIBILITY

Masters (1993) states that Lawyers:

"are reluctant to accept that free will can be diverted by anything less than severe and easily recognisable illness. Doctors on the other hand, are equally reluctant to admit that freedom of choice can escape from the restraints of biochemical makeup or psychological influence."

Lord Hale stated in 1736 that "where there is a total defect of understanding, there is no free act of the will". Masters (1993) states that while Dahlmer when he was involved in this activity he didn't have a mental illness there is no doubt he did have a mental disorder called Autistic Psychopathy. Nevertheless this differentiation between mental illness and mental disorder is important. The idea of mental illness is a rather outdated concept and now we use the phrase mental disorder. There is also decreasing evidence of a lack of differentiation between so-called mental disorders and personality disorders. There are underlying biochemistry in both. In the past "psychopathic personality" did not carry any aetiological explanation. It does:

> "Mental illness could be used as an insanity defence but personality disorder not. I think that the McNaughten rule points out that "a criminal is not to be held responsible if, by reason of a disease of the mind, he does not know the nature and quality of his acts, or does not know that they are wrong".(Masters, 1993)

Masters (1993) states clearly that Dahlmer knew this but he could not stop himself, nevertheless he was under an overwhelming impulse. He had a mental disability Criminal Autistic Psychopathy. According to Masters:

> "a man could know right from wrong would either be deficient in emotional appreciation that what he did was wrong or be unable to control his behaviour because his unlawful act was the product of mental disease or mental defect."

Certainly Dahlmer had a mental defect (Criminal Autistic Psychopathy) and was unable to control his behaviour.

The America Law Institute states that

> "A person is not responsible for criminal conduct if at the time of such conduct as a result of mental disease or defect he lacks substantial capacity either to appreciate the wrongfulness of his conduct or to conform his conduct to the requirements of the law."

The American Psychiatric Association (1982) states that "the line between an irresistible impulse and an impulse not resisted is probably no sharper than that between twilight and dusk".

According to Kenneth Smale in a Postscript to Masters book on Dahlmer, Dahlmer did want to find that "there was something not part of him (a disease) that made him want to commit his crimes" In a way he was partly right and this was Criminal Autistic Psychopathy, which is a developmental disorder. It is clear he couldn't control his killing behaviour and if released would do the same again. In terms of the Wisconsin statutes in relation to insanity "a person is not responsible for criminal conduct if at the time of such conduct as a result of mental disease or defect he lacked substantial capacity to appreciate the wrongfulness of his conduct or conform his conduct to the requirements of the law" He knew it was wrong but couldn't control it.

Brittain (1970) states that sometimes they can respond well to the structured prison situation and be good prisoners "given the opportunity the sadistic murderer is likely to murder again and he knows this". Jeffrey Dahlmer's father said that "as a scientist, I further wonder if this potential for great evil also resides deep in the blood".

Dahlmer did know right from wrong but he could not control the impulse therefore he had diminished responsibility. He had clearly lost control of his impulses. While very early identification might lend to treatment in early life prior to serial killing once the serial killing has started the prognosis is very poor. It was a compulsive addictive behaviour. At the end it had taken over his life.

Chapter 13

CASE HISTORIES OF MALE SERIAL KILLERS AND CRIMINAL AUTISTIC PYSCOPATHY

ALBERT DE SALVO: THE BOSTON STRANGLER

According to Leyton (1989), De Salvo had "murdered 13 women and sexually assaulted nearly 1000, which, in fact, seems a likely estimate"

Frank (1967) stated that around "the necks of the victims were knotted nylon stockings or other articles of their apparel. Each woman had been sexually molested or assaulted. No clues were found; nothing had been stolen; there was no discernable motive. The victims were, so far as could be determined, modest, inconspicuous, almost anonymous women, leading blameless lives". De Salvo confessed in great detail after being caught.

Background

De Salvo said he had a deprived childhood and was ill treated by his father. There was a lack of food in the home and much domestic violence. His father was also a criminal and interpersonally violent. His parents were divorced. Albert spent time in the army and in the military police. He abused a 9-year-old girl while in the army. He was court-martialled there. He refused to obey orders (Leyton, 1980). Serial killers often have some form of involvement with the police. Albert was always a loner and a poor mixer in general. He had a miserable time at school. He began shoplifting even in the pre-school period. He was a voyeur and killed cats as a child. He was probably of average intelligence and worked as a carpenter's helper.

Leyton (1980) notes that he had a very traumatic childhood. Indeed "his father sold him and his sister as slaves to a farmer" He was a very rejected child. He stole also as a young person. He was put in to a reform school, which had only the effect of training him more in criminal activities. He also did a considerable amount of breaking and entering. He was an immature personality and dependent on his wife. When his wife had a very difficult pregnancy it put her off sex. Persons with Criminal Autistic Psychopathy often blame others for their problems. He blamed his wife.

Sexuality

He had an extremely high sex drive and was annoyed when sexually rejected by his wife. This was a triggering factor for some of his sexual behaviour. He had sexually identity diffusion and worked as a "rent boy" (Leyton, 1989).

Cawthorne (2002) states that he was called the "Measuring Man" because of going around to young ladies and measuring them and saying that he was looking for people to do modelling in an agency. He claimed he assaulted about 1,000 women. They were of a variety of ages. He would then go home and have his dinner with the family. He loved to demean girls. He received a diagnosis of Sociopathic Personality for carrying out this kind of activity. He convinced the Judge to be lenient with him and persons like this are often very persuasive.

Killing

Leyton (1989) describes that De Salvo's first attempt at murdering a woman was unsuccessful, because he looked at himself in the mirror and this made him realise what he was doing and he ran away. Later that month, he tried to kill again and was successful. This was in 1962. He pretended he was a maintenance man and women would let him into their apartment and then he would kill them. After the killing he would mess up the apartments. As he progressed with the killings, he engaged in sexual assaults and also putting foreign objects into the women's vaginas. He tended to strangle his victims. Occasionally he did feel guilt, and it is not true to say that all serial killers or all persons with Criminal Autistic Psychopathy have zero guilt. They have a very diminished capacity for guilt and diminished capacity for empathy, but it is not always absent. There is great heterogeneity.

De Salvo was a great confessor of his activities. He also tended to discuss his killings in the third person, which is typical of Criminal Autistic Psychopathy. His youngest victim was 20 years and oldest 85 years of age.

Frank (1967) states that De Salvo left "his victims in obscene positions, as if deliberately to debase and degrade them". At one of the murders he left a note for the police "Happy New Year!" He could act as a pseudo-normal man at work. He was a Jekyll and Hyde figure. Killing was a self-esteem regulator for him and made him feel important and in control. His great aim was to be talked about as a celebrity. He boasted about his activities and wanted to be important. It took the police quite a while to believe that he was the Boston Strangler and he was spending his time trying to convince them giving them more and more details. He had a massive memory. The women were random and anonymous figures to him. Before he was finally caught, "he had been under their noses (police) all the time! More, the police and the Courts had actually had their hands on him several times before" This is quite typical as well of Criminal Autistic Psychopathy . He took the police around to show them the apartments where his victims had lived. The British Psychiatrist William Sergeant assessed him. But it did seem to me that he was not able to throw much light on the case. He did not have Schizophrenia, but criminal Autistic Psychopathy.

His life ended when he was killed in prison during an episode of interpersonal contact with another prisoner.

ED GEIN

Ed Gein was a savage serial killer born over one hundred years ago in the United States. He died of natural causes in 1984. Both his father and mother were very strange persons and appear to have had Asperger's syndrome traits. His father was an aggressive, moody, introverted figure, while his mother was a bible lover and religious zealot. She regarded most women as prostitutes to be kept clear of and she had a horror of sex (which was only for producing children) and was severely harsh on her two sons in relation to masturbation.

As with most persons with Criminal Autistic Psychopathy, Ed Gein was bullied in his earlier life. He showed very odd, eccentric, non-verbal behaviour especially in relation to his face when he would break out in inappropriate laughter. He was a great reader. He had major problems with empathy and reciprocal social relationships. It is not beyond the bounds of possibility that he killed his brother, as he was the last one to see him alive.

Gein's behaviour with the bodies he killed was very similar to Jeffrey Dahlmer. He was a necrophiliac and operated in graveyards to acquire skulls etc. He made clothes for himself out of people, e.g. skin etc. Like Irma Grese, the female killer, he made lampshades out of their skin. He mutilated the bodies and used skulls to make soup bowls. There was probably also some cannibalism. It is not clear how many people he killed. He appears to have been a transsexual and wanted a conversion to the female sex. He influenced many Hollywood movies including *Psycho, The Texas Chainsaw Massacre, The Silence of the Lambs, In the Light of the Moon,* and *House of 1000 corpses.*

GILLES DE RAIS

Gilles de Rais was described as "the world's wickedness man" (Wolf, 1980). He showed the greatest savagery and cruelty in his behaviour. Like many people with Criminal Autistic Psychopathy he was of a mystical bent and a churchgoer. Wolf notes that he was both cruel and a mystic and his crimes make one think about "the religious greatness of the damned; genius as disease, disease as genius…where saint and criminal become one". This quotation is from Thomas Mann "*Dostoyevski – Within Limits*" in the Thomas Mann Reader Ed. Walter Angell. There was this split in his personality between the churchgoer and the sadistic killer.

Dostoevsky's fictional man in his novel, *Stavrogin's Confession,* states a number of sentiments which Gilles de Rais could have experienced that:

> "every unusually disgraceful, utterly degrading, dastardly, and above all, ridiculous situation, in which I ever happened to be in my life always roused in me, side by side with extreme anger, and incredible delight . . If I stole, I would feel, while committing the theft, a rapture from the consciousness of the depth of my vileness. It was not the vileness that I loved (here my mind was perfectly sound), but I enjoyed the rapture from the tormenting consciousness of the baseness."

According to Wolf (1980), he was also described as "the beast of extermination" and "the devourer of Machecoul (a place name) – the poor fool who tried to catch God and Satan in the same net". For Leonard Wolf, serial killing is a kind of rage that completely takes over the individual and for which they have no control over it. In *The Black Cat*, Edgar Allan Poe talks about "the spirit of perverseness . . . (as) one of the primitive impulses of the human heart, one of the indivisible primary faculties, or sentiments, which give direction to the character of man" Edgar Allan Poe. The Black Cat in complete work of Edgar Allan Poe. It is interesting that Poe and Dostoyevski both had Autistic Psychopathy (Asperger's Syndrome).

Personal History

Gilles de Rais was born in 1404 and came from an extremely rich ruling family. Thomas Mann also wrote in the same book that he was "a gifted normal intellect who (moves upwards to icy, abnormal spheres of comprehension and moral isolation); to a frightful, criminal degree of knowingness" He was a Latin scholar. He had an artistic temperament. He was very interested in music. He was also a man of science and the arts. He recognised no limits.

Schneider (1964) wrote "there is no true work of art in which the demon is not a collaborator . . the artist cannot succeed without the aid of god's monkey" He was a great collector. He had an interest in alchemy and Satanism. He sold things for much less than he bought them like William Hearst the great American newspaper tycoon and collector who also had Autistic Psychopathy.

He lost his father in 1415 in a hunting accident and his mother a short time later. He was then reared by Jean de Craon who according to George Bataille "thought Gilles to believe himself above the law". (George Bataille, 1965).).

Attachment theory psychology would try to explain all his behaviour as due to early attachment relationships. This is absurd.

Gilles worked extremely hard to become a Knight, deal with the armour, and deal with the style of warfare practised at the time. He engaged in homosexuality. Gilles then married a close relative. On the battlefield Gilles enjoyed murder and carnage. He loved hanging people.

Gilles did anything he wanted to do. He was amoral. Wolf (1980) compares him to other nasty people from history fictional and historical including Dr. Moro in Welles novel, Lady MacBeth, and Iago from Shakespeare as well as Richard III who was a real historical figure and about whom Shakespeare wrote a play.

Personal History and Characteristics

Gilles was a novelty seeker and a sensation seeker. He was perverse. He was an evil man. Gilles had little interest in heterosexual relations but did engage with his wife for the sake of having an heir. This did occur. At the same time he was on the road of a "torturer / murderer" (Wolf, 1980). They then separated. She married again when Gilles was executed. Gilles remained emotionally immature. He wanted instant gratification. He moved between "the orgy and the altar" (Wolf, 1980). He showed extreme perversion. He loved "flavoured foods" (Wolf, 1980). (This issue of flavoured food is from Georges Bataille La proc de Gilles de Rais). He loved to go beyond the limits, to go too far. He liked alcohol. He did everything to excess. He suffered from depression. He had "the sexual energies of a satyr" (Wolf, 1980).

Gilles showed a great deal of restlessness. He was ultimately extremely self-destructive. He was sadistic, he was narcissistic, he spent extravagantly and wastefully, and he was exhibitionistic in the way he spent. He paid excessively for what he bought. He was a shopaholic. He showed poor reality testing, was grandiose, and he was a child abuser. He was extremely narcissistic. He was self-destructive and masochistic as well as vengeful and ritualistic.

He got more perverse and worse as he got older. He behaved as if he was omnipotent. At times he seemed to have difficulty separating fact from fiction. He engaged in 8 to 14 years of child homicide. He found the killing orgasmic. He became addicted to killing He then mixed this with Satanism. He killed between 141 and 800 according to Wolf.

Murdering Children

Morrison and Goldberg (2004) state that de Rais sent his servants to town "to search out the prettiest children, mostly boys (although a few girls were gathered up as well). His lackeys lied to parents, sometimes saying the great, heroic baron was going to send their sons and daughters away for a proper education". De Rais "revelled in children's panic".

He would hang the children and they would pass out and then he would revive them and hug them. Then, he would cut a vein in the neck of the child and "began to masturbate as the blood spurted wildly from every waning heartbeat. De Rais enjoyed slicing open the belly of a child and masturbating until he climaxed into it" (Morrison and Goldberg, 2004). His valet stated that the killings were "sometimes beheading or decapitating them, sometimes cutting their throats, sometimes dismembering them, and sometimes breaking their necks with a cudgel" (Morrison and Goldberg, 2004). He was hanged for the murder of 140 children. "De Rais began to kill once his closest relative had passed on. It was similar to Ed Gein, in that Gein began killing after his mother died and Richard Macek began his rampage after his father died" (Morrison and Goldberg, 2004). There was some trigger factor here.

Wolf (1980) stated that Dostoyevski wrote in the *Brothers Karamazov* "it is characteristic of many people, this love of torturing children, and children are only. Its just their defencelessness that tempts the tormentor, angelic confidence of the child who has no refuge and no appeal, that sets his vile blood on fire" Wolf notes that in relation to the children he might have been attracted to "the image, in the androgynous bodies of the children, of the androgynous gender in her boys clothing" (Wolf, 1980). He went from the church to the murder chamber. He used to get children by whatever means was necessary. Some were beggar children. They were all vulnerable. The parents suffered greatly on losing their children. Gilles premeditated his killing and only chose good-looking children. He was quite seductive to them initially and then the nasty bit came.

JOAN OF ARC AND GILLES DE RAIS

Gilles linked up with Joan of Arc which was unusual but there may have been some idiosyncrasy in both their personalities that attracted each other, i.e. that they both had Asperger's Syndrome Autistic Psychopathy of different forms. Gilles in battle was very courageous.

Wolf (1980) points out that it appears that "Gilles had been playing the double roles of Jan's friend and la Tremoilles spy". He abandoned Joan of Arc immediately after she was captured. It appeared that he just did not care.

GRAHAM YOUNG

George Orwell wrote in the *Decline of the English Murder* (1946) that "you never seem to get a good murder these days" (Holden, 1995). Orwell was wrong.

Graham Young was a serial killer. He poisoned his victims. He was an experimental criminal Autistic Psychopath.

Background

Graham Young's father was "a withdrawn and far from self-sufficient man" (Anthony Holden, 1995). His stepmother was Irish and was called Molly. Graham was an autodictat. He read a great detail and was highly intelligent. He studied what interested him, rather than the regular school curriculum. He was shy and hypersensitive as a child. He was also socially awkward and also always related poorly to children his own age.. He did not know how to handle strangers as a child. He could get on better with adults. As a child he would kick over "old ladies' shopping bags, teasing neighbours pets" etc. He was eccentric and had very odd interests for a child. He said he would become a famous poisoner. He started by fantasying killing. He was able to relate to a couple of peers who had the same interests as himself. He was also interested in killing animals and doing autopsies on them (Holden, 1995).

Graham Young (Emsley, 2005) as a child showed "excessive rocking to-and-fro in his cot". He had poor sleep patterns. He was a "withdrawn little boy". He was fascinated by "model aeroplanes". He was "fat and awkward" as well as being "withdrawn and secretive". His nickname was "Pudding" in the family. He was fascinated with murder by poison and also by "occult and black magic, and the Nazis". He was fascinated by chemical elements and is supposed to have poisoned his family cat. He was also fascinated by fire. He showed poor school performance. The students in his school called him the "Mad Professor". Students with Asperger's syndrome are often called professors. He told the students "of his ambition to become a famous poisoner" He was seen by a Child Psychiatrist who diagnosed psychopathy, which was correct, but Criminal Autistic Psychopathy would even have been more correct nowadays. In the Ashford Remand Centre he attempted suicide (Emsley, 2005).

His school became concerned because of his unusual interests and because bottles of poison were found in his desk. He was seen by a Child Psychiatrist who reported his activity to the police. He was arrested. He was one of the youngest people to go to Broadmoor. His lack of conscience was noted when he went into the Ashford Remand Centre (Holden, 1995).

Profile

He was a loner, narcissistic, egocentric, grandiose, and exhibitionistic. He was very excited and indeed was addicted to killing. He had a massive memory. He had "one or two odd traits, such as cleaning his teeth every time he ate anything and he carried a toothbrush around with him for this purpose. He was also fanatical about killing insects" (Emsley, 2005).

Narrow Interest

Graham was very interested in poisons and murder. He was also fascinated by the occult and the Nazis. He liked the paraphernalia of killing and used to draw the paraphernalia of killing i.e., syringes, poisons, images of people being hanged etc. (Holden, 1995).

He wanted to get training in the police "Forensic Science Laboratory" and indeed with the "Pharmaceutical Society's Training Scheme" (Holden, 1995).

Young suggested that the IRA should be eliminated in the way that the Jews were eliminated in the Warsaw ghetto by Hitler. People found him emotionless (Holden, 1995).

As well as describing himself as Frankenstein, he was also fascinated by Dracula. He admired two killers in particular - Dr. Edward Pritchard and also the killer Palmer. His great interest was toxicology. Indeed his personality was similar to Pritchard's - being narcissistic, egocentric, grandiose, and exhibitionistic. He would take some of his poison around with him, e.g. antimony. It was a kind of almost comfort to him or a kind of autistic object (Holden, 1995). Like many persons with these criminal interests, Young had an interest in joining the police.

Control, Language, and Social Relationships

Young was controlling and dominating in communication and spoke in monologues. He had very poor reciprocal social relationships. He lacked remorse.

Again in Broadmoor, he tended to relate poorly to other inmates and was seen as grandiose and narcissistic. He was not popular with other inmates. He showed sexual identity diffusion and did not have a clear heterosexual identity. Neither did he have a homosexual identity. In Broadmoor, the nurses were quite worried about Young's progress and realised his dangerousness. They noted that he was living "in a fantasy world" (Holden, 1995). They found it hard to have meaningful relationships with him. He was only interested in discussing his toxicology.

At his trial, he reminds one of Ted Bundy because of his linguistic interchanges with both the prosecuting and defensive counsels. He wanted a long drawn out trial.

It is likely that he probably poisoned somebody and killed in Broadmoor, although it has not been definitively proven that it was he who did it. The rumour was that he used cyanide.

Professionals' Involvement

Graham was seen by Dr. Christopher Fish who noted his poor prognosis and stated that it was "extremely likely" that if he was at liberty that he will repeat the poisoning (Holden, 1995). He was also seen by Dr. James Cameron, a Psychiatrist at The Maudsley Hospital in London, who felt that he was "far too dangerous to be even in that Hospital" (Holden, 1995). These were very accurate assessments.

Nevertheless the major Psychiatrists were Dr. Patrick McGrath and Dr. Edgar Udwin, a Jewish Psychiatrist.

After the first year in Broadmoor, Dr. Udwin was "predicting a remarkably early release" (Holden, 1995). Other inmates said that he was "McGrath's blue-eyed boy" (Holden, 1995). Dr. McGrath was a most distinguished British psychiatrist. Udwin and McGrath consulted regularly about the boy who was fast becoming their star patient" (Holden, 1995). He had autistic charm.

In 1970, Dr. Udwin stated that "he is no longer a danger to others" (Holden, 1995). At the same time, Young described himself as "Frankenstein". Dr. Udwin had been praised in the press as "Broadmoor's Hero Doctor" The nurses were clear that Young intended to poison again if he was let out. He wanted to be a famous killer/poisoner (Holden, 1995). The nurses were right.

At around 15 years of age, he spent a few years in Broadmoor and was released because he was "cured" (Holden, 1995). "The two men responsible for recommending Graham's rehabilitation were Dr. Patrick McGrath, Medical Superintendent and Dr. Edgar Udwin, who was his personal psychiatrist". He was not rehabilitated. Dr. McGrath "appointed Graham a staff tea-boy" This was not a successful appointment as Young put "Harpic lavatory cleaner in the tea one day". After his release, he began killing again. In 1971, Dr. Udwin stated that he had "made an extremely full recovery" (Holden, 1995). Holden also states that "Dr. Udwin's part in Young's release had been dangerously autonomous". He had not recovered which was indeed the nurses' view.

Poisoning and Killing History

Graham was a random killer. He killed people whom he came across by accident. It was the excitement of the experiment that interested him and watching them die. Poisoning is what gave a buzz to his life and without it he would become depressed. Like other persons with Criminal Autistic Psychopathy, when taken into custody at this time he confessed everything. He was addicted to poisoning and killing. He was incapable of stopping it. This was all known at his first arrest. Most of his poisoning involved the putting of poisons into tea. He used antimony and also thallium. He used to joke about putting poison in people's tea. It was no joke!

When he was released, he started working in a factory and began to poison people and killed people again. He even boasted how easy it was to produce physical symptoms in a person through poisoning and that the person would be diagnosed with a typical physical illness. The people in the factory were baffled by the illness and death. They thought about radiation, they also thought about poisoning, and they thought about viruses. Nevertheless they were not able to pin down anything. At a staff meeting consider these events, Young was extremely vocal and particularly pushed the poisoning issue. People realised that the illnesses had started when Young had joined the staff. They mentioned their suspicions to the police who made a raid and found all his equipment. This led to his arrest. He told them about a pharmaceutical substance that would counter the poisoning. They also found his diary which listed a great deal about the killings. Later he described the diary as a work of fiction and that he was interested in writing. He asked his interogators if they had read the *Ballad of Reading Gaol*? He recited the beginning of it: "Yet each man kills the thing he loves, by each let this be heard" (Holden, 1995). He wanted a long drawn out trial and wanted the media attention of the trial so he could have his moment in the limelight.

He denied everything during the court case and said in reply to a question "I do not feel particularly calm, Mr. Leonard, but I am not a person who manifests a great amount of emotion" (Holden, 1995). This is a feature of Criminal Autistic Psychopathy. He showed no emotion when he was sentenced to life imprisonment. He also went to prison rather than back to Broadmoor and in his controlling fashion he achieved this himself. He died of a heart attack in 1990 in prison.

HARVEY GLATMAN

Harvey Glatman (Newton 1998) was a shy loner. He was an outsider. He was obsessed with having power and control of women. He was extremely ambivalent about women. His main interest was domination, control, power, and rape. The killing was incidental to his wish to make sure that the woman did not tell the police about him. His instrument was a section of rope that he carried around with him. He strangled people with it. He took souvenirs from his victims e.g. undergarments. He had massive superego lacunae or conscience deficits. Nevertheless, he was not completely without conscience and would feel guilt after a killing. He took photographs of women after he had them tied up. These photographs gave him great pleasure in the period after the killing.

Background

His mother noticed "instances of strange behaviour" by him in the preschool period. She said he "tied a string around his penis, placed the loose end in a drawer, and then leaned back against the string" (Newton, 1998).

Serial killers tend to be closer to mothers and more distant from fathers. They are often compulsive masturbators, are often fetishistic and voyeuristic. Newton (1998) points out that as a child Harvey indulged in "bondage verging on masochism" that is "genital ligation and self-inflicted pain" in the preschool period. At puberty he use to "tie a rope around his neck, get in the bathtub, run the rope's free end around a crossbar on the drain, and pull it tight until he climaxed in a breathless rush" (Newton, 1998). He would at other times put the rope around the rafters – autoerotic asphyxia – to heighten his orgasm. This can lead to accidental death. It is an autistic novelty seeking or sensation seeking strategy. It is a very addictive phenomenon. With him you see the multiple perversions that often accompany serial killers.

Harvey, in his multiple IQ tests, showed superior intelligence. He was particularly good at reading, arithmetic and music, as well as taking photographs. He was interested in engineering and became a radio and TV repairman. He was a hypersensitive boy. He had a very unstable work record. He wanted to be a celebrity – a very famous man and was quite narcissistic. He first got excitement from breaking and entering homes and stealing. Then he moved on to raping women, photographing them when he had tied them up with rope, and then killing them. His mother felt he should have had a leucotomy. He received all the standard psychiatric diagnoses at the time, e.g. schizophrenia, psychopathy, and sexual deviation. Schizophrenia was a diagnosis that was used very loosely in America at that time. He never had schizophrenia. Criminal Autistic Psychopathy would have been a more accurate diagnosis than Psychopathic Personality.

In 1948, he entered Sing Sing Prison. He studied radio engineering there. The structure of the prison suited him. He also acted as librarian there. Dr. Franklin E. Baugh noted that he thought in "clichés and stereotypes" This is not uncommonly the language of criminal Autistic Psychopaths and is an autistic narrative. He blamed others for his problems and showed paranoid anxiety. He could not deal with reciprocal social relationships. He found social relationships unrewarding. He had an emotionally immature personality. He had a lot of repressed anger. He had sexual identify diffusion and had a very poor sense of self – sexual and non-sexual. He saw himself as an outsider and that he was one of life's outsiders. He was very narcissistic and wanted to be admired but did not get it or do things to get it. His mother was non-judgemental and accepting of him. It is hardly surprising because of his poor social skills, poor capacity for empathy that people did not seek him out or warm to him. He had a general feeling of being hurt and not accepted by other human beings. When out of prison he would drift without employment for years at a time. He often suffered from depression and suicidal ideas. He was very sensitive to smell and noise. He could be contemptuous of bosses and other workers. He related poorly in the work situation. He was a visual thinker.

For most serial killers there is quite a gap between the first and second killing. Then the gap reduces for the killing thrill is required more frequently. Harvey liked "fooling" the police. Harvey also threatened people with a gun before raping them. Newton (1998) noted Harvey's "quirks". After the killing the photographs of the women he killed were used for masturbatory purposes. This type of satisfaction would begin to wear off. He would feel the tension building up in himself and the need to rape again. He would go looking for a victim e.g. in the small ads or elsewhere. He had piercing eyes something that is often seen in persons with Autistic Psychopathy. The press described him as "owl-eyed" (Page 193). On the last attempt at rape the woman challenged him, got out of the car, and on to a road and a policeman saw her shouting and struggling and arrested Harvey. He confessed immediately with a very meticulous, detailed narrative. This is typical of Criminal Autistic Psychopathy. In Prison he hated being watched and it upset him greatly. He insisted on the death penalty another form of control. He wanted to take the decision out of his Solicitors hands. Harvey was the classic Jekyll and Hyde type of person.

William Lavelle a Probation Officer interviewed mother and was told that he would even "walk across the street to avoid females" What he was looking for was companionship. He also believed he could no longer control his desires to rape, dominate and control women. This was the only kind of sexual satisfaction he felt he was capable of achieving. He was a great reader as persons with Autistic Psychopathy often are.

A psychologist W. A. Drummond (Newton, 1998) noted his impulsivity, poor control of temper, moodiness, drifting lifestyle, no friendships, contempt for people of lesser ability than him, and that he wanted an operation to "reduce his hearing but about 90%" and that he had a Schizoid Personality a diagnosis that was used in the past for Autistic Psychopathy. Persons with Autistic Psychopathy often have very acute hearing, which can be upsetting to them. They experience sensory overload. Clearly using the rope was a sexualised behaviour for him that excited him. At the end Harvey blamed the lack of treatment he received growing up for his problems – blaming others – and did not show guilt for his killings. Like many persons with Autistic Psychopathy he had a quirky sense of humour (Lyons and Fitzgerald, 2004) and called his last meal the "gas chamber special". He was executed.

ADOLF HITLER HAD AUTISTIC PSYCHOPATHY

The personality of Adolf Hitler has puzzled people for almost 100 years. Everyone who knew him found him an enigma. Indeed Otto Wagener who was chief of the SA (Sturmabteilung: Storm Troop) saw Hitler's character as "something foreign and diabolical. Hitler remained for him altogether a puzzle" (Kershaw, 1998). He was regarded as being "distinctly odd" (Kershaw, 1998). A phrase from Winston Churchill could be very usefully applied to Hitler. The phrase was "a riddle wrapped in a mystery inside an enigma" (Kershaw, 1998).

Firstly, his personal and family history will be examined. Klara Polzl was his mother. Klara's wedding took place at 6.00 a.m. in the morning and she only had the most perfunctory celebration after which her new husband went immediately back to his customs post. According to the family doctor Eduard Bloch, Klara was an unremarkable woman. Hitler's mother's life was not easy with the deaths of her three first children and then being married to an unempathetic, domineering and dictatorial husband aggravated her sorrows. It is hardly surprising that she spoiled and was overprotective of her son Adolf. Indeed, the family doctor Dr. Bloch stated that he was very attached to her. Excessive attachment to mother is common in persons with Asperger's syndrome. Adolf Hitler carried his mother's picture to his death.

Hitler's father, Alois, was a child born outside of marriage of Marianna Schicklgruber daughter of a poor small holder. Alois was the first "social climber in the family" (Kershaw, 1998). Despite limited education, he became a customs inspector Alois was a local petty public servant. He was an obsessional nitpicker. He had a very limited personality. He probably had autistic traits. He had very poor control of his temper and was quite unpredictable in relation to his temper. He took very little interest in the rearing of his family and was happier outside the family than inside. His passion was for looking after bees. He showed no emotional warmth to any one including Adolf. Hitler's sister Paula stated that "Adolf challenged their father to extreme harshness and he use to get a sound trashing everyday" and indeed Hitler himself stated in the 1940s that "his father had sudden bursts of temper and would then immediately hit out" (Kershaw, 1998). It is hardly surprising that Hitler's mother did the best she could to protect Adolf from father's savage attacks.

As a pre-schooler, Hitler showed poor emotional control and got into rages if he could not have everything the way he wanted it. He then went to a Real Schule, which focussed on science and technical studies. He had "no close friends at school; nor did he seek any"

(Kershaw, 1998). He was a rather lazy and unsatisfactory student. He was unable to accommodate himself to the school discipline and was regarded as being dictatorial, controlling, and obsessional. He grew into a lazy aimless teenager. He was ultimately a failure at school and often feigned illness, which is not untypical in persons with Asperger's syndrome He fantasised a great deal about becoming a great artist and sat up late at night while sleeping late in the morning. He became infatuated with a girl who did not know even of his existence and she was called Stephanie (Kershaw, 1998). This is not uncommon in persons with Asperger's Syndrome.

The family doctor Dr. Bloch described Hitler as a fragile loner who was anxious about his mother. He failed in the examination to get into the Academy of Fine Arts in Vienna and began to develop "a drifting existence in an egoistic fantasy-world" (Kershaw, 1998). He lived in Vienna from 1908 to 1913 being aged 18 when he arrived there and basically drifted there. He was obsessed with monumental grandiose plans. He was extremely narcissistic. He always had an interest in architecture and sketched Viennese buildings. Visual impact was very important to him. He clearly had a formidable memory but he used this simply to confirm in his reading already existing opinions (Kershaw, 1998).

In 1909 in Vienna, he lived either rough or slept in cheap lodgings. He was an unhygienic individual, very poorly dressed and clearly this 20 year old was close to skid row with all other homeless alcoholics. Even in the rooms of the men's homes that he stayed in, he was regarded as eccentric. He gradually developed a conspiracy theory about Jews and linked Jews with every perceived evil (Kershaw, 1998). In one house that he stayed in for two years in Vienna, he did not have a single visitor during all that time. He was clearly a loner. In a way he was rescued by the 1st World War, and joined up the army, which became his place of refuge. He was a dispatch runner during the War and was decorated with medals. After the war he returned to Munich, and became a member of the German Workers Party and began his rise basically as a "mob orator" (Kershaw, 1998). Then followed his relatively rapid rise to become leader of the German nation, which inevitably lead to the 2nd World War and to his death by suicide.

Criminal Autistic Psychopathy

What is the evidence for his Autistic Psychopathy? Well, he showed a gross lack of normal social integration. As Kershaw (1998) pointed out Hitler had an "innate secretiveness, an emptiness of personal relations, an unbureaucratic style" and stirred up adulation and hatred. He had autistic charisma and lacked a rounded personality and was an outsider. Basically he had no real relationships with most people, with the possible exception of his mother, and was in the privileged position of a self-preoccupied loner. He had no close friends.

He had a deep disgust and repugnance of sexual activity and was repelled by homosexuality. He recoiled from close relationships and had an inability to "forge genuine friendship" and showed an enormous emptiness in his human relations (Kershaw, 1998). His lectures to people in the Men's Homes in Vienna were really monologues and invited no reciprocity. He lacked the capacity for intimacy and also for reciprocity in social relationships having a capacity for social isolation.

In Vienna he was described as being distant, self-contained, withdrawn and without friends (Kershaw, 1998). In his Munich period before the 1st World War, he would simply harangue the people around him, rather than try and communicate with them in a reciprocal way. While in the army his colleagues noted that he was eccentric and socially isolated, but was a great reader. To his fellow soldiers in the 1st World War, he seemed an eccentric alien without humour and the nearest he got to showing any affection was to his dog. Another phrase that his comrades in arms used about him was that he was strange and it was clear that he had no capacity for any interpersonal feeling.

After the 1st World War, he stood out as a very powerful person when he spoke as a "mob orator", but was extremely diffident, ill at ease, socially awkward and uncertain with small groups of individuals. He was not a people person and despised the human race. His colleagues regarded him as a remote figure - an obsessive who was extremely boring and engaged in odd monologues. He would spend the afternoon in Café Heck in Munich where his cronies and admirers would listen to his repetitive boring dialogue about the war. In addition, Kershaw (1998) reports that there was "something other-worldly about Hitler and he had a lack of knowledge of human beings and with it a lack of sound judgement of them" and indeed that he lived without "any bonds to another human being" During his lifetime, he only took a slight interest in a couple of women. One was Geli who effectively became his prisoner, and not surprisingly she said of him "my uncle is a monster" and completed suicide. His second relationship was with Eva Braun who also attempted suicide and died with him in the bunker.

All Absorbing Narrow Interest

He had an all-absorbing narrow interest in power, a hatred of the Jews, and interest in architecture. All his speeches were extremely repetitive based on the narrow themes of hatred of the Jews and how Germany had been abused after the 1st World War. He spent a great deal of time with Albert Speer, examining architectural plans and this remained a major focus throughout his life. His other major interest was in the music of Wagner. He had a rigid one track mind.

Hitler's greatest interest was clearly being able to control and exert power over people. His ability to achieve this control and power was clearly extraordinary and "he was able to extend his power until it became absolute, until field marshals were prepared to obey without question the orders of a former corporal, until highly skilled professionals and clever minds in all walks of life were ready to pay uncritical obedience to an autodidact" (Kershaw, 1998). He became a dictator who felt he was always right. He had absolute control of the Government when he came into power and was "largely detached from any formal machinery of Government" (Kershaw, 1998).

Non-Verbal Aspects of Communication

He showed impairment in the non-verbal aspects of communication. During the 1st World War, other soldiers noted him sitting at the periphery of groups with minimal non-verbal expression. They also noticed that he had "the look of the Monk" It was clear that his quirky behaviour singled him out from the rest of the group and he was regarded as being "distinctly odd" (Kershaw, 1998). He was physically awkward. In Munich at that time, he could be seen travelling around "in his gangster and trench coat" with his dog whip. His strangeness interested people. Even though he was regarded as being odd he had curiosity value.

Speech and Language Problems

As regards speech and language problems, he certainly did not use language for the purpose of interchange with others, but only for the purpose of dominating others. He endlessly engaged in long winded pedantic speeches. He had an odd prosody, but of course this was very powerful. Indeed when Anton Drexler the leader of the DAP (Deutsche Arbeiter Partei – German Workers' Party) heard him first speak in September 1919 he stated that "goodness, he has got a gob. We could use him" (Kershaw, 1998). He was also described as being "a born agitator in spite of a voice sometimes broken and not infrequently croaking" (Kershaw, 1998).

Discussion

Adolf Hitler does meet the criteria for Criminal Autistic Psychopathy as described by Hans Asperger (1944). It was this combination of a person with autistic psychopathy and a nation in turmoil after the 1st World War, even though this nation was modern, cultured, and technologically advanced. He sent millions of Jews and others to their deaths in the Holocaust. Nevertheless, he was not a sadistic serial killer in the sense of this book. Clearly, Hitler's extremely poor relationship with his father was a negative factor in his development but if he did not have Criminal Autistic Psychopathy, his good relationship with his mother should have protected him and normally does.

Unfortunately good mothering cannot cure Criminal Autistic Psychopathy. It would appear that his father also had autistic psychopathy and that this was transmitted genetically to him. Probably in the history of the world, there has never been such a devastating interaction between an individual with severe psychopathology and a nation in turmoil looking for a saviour.

JEFFREY DAHLMER

Background

Jeffrey Dahlmer was a serial killer who later murdered himself. He made a full confession when caught, of many murders that the police knew nothing about which is typical of persons with Criminal Autistic Psychopathy. He mentioned 16 murders and that six of the murders were very recent. He liked to keep many of the heads at least for a short period of time. He mentioned that his first murder happened in 1978. This interview with police took place in July 1991.

Nevertheless his murder tally was 17 at the end of his killing career. He killed a number in his grandmother's house. Others, he killed in a hotel room and in his flat. He thought of his murderous activities in terms of a murder lust (Masters, 1993).

Lionel Dahlmer (1995) points out "it was not the suffering of his victims that had delighted and aroused Dahlmer. It was their deaths and dismemberments".

Jeffrey suffered a lot from infections in his early life, which may have been due to a reduced autoimmune system. This is common in Autistic Psychopathy.

Jeffrey was fascinated as a child by "the gutted fish" when he was fishing with father. He was fascinated by "the power of old bones like little sticks" (Dahlmer, 1995). His father remembered Jeffrey killing tadpoles as a child.

Jeffrey loved animal's bones and played with them (Masters, 1993). He was fascinated by animals and insects (Masters, 1993). In his childhood, he was most interested in dinosaurs and was very much a collector.

He collected animal skeletons. He had an animal graveyard where he buried animals. One of the items he collected as a small boy was a skull of a pig. He became obsessed with dead animals and collecting animals that were killed on the roads. He dissected them and was always fascinated by the insides of both animals and humans. He wanted to know how the animal worked. He saw dead animals as a kind of robotic figures where he could work out their mechanisms of action by dissecting them.

In general, as one finds with persons with Criminal Autistic Psychopathy, he related better to animals than humans. He was an avid book reader.

Hi father said, "he was a lonely child with poor social interaction not interested in sports". He said that Jeffrey liked:

> "Games whose rules were highly defined and non-confrontational, games full of repetitious actions, particularly those that were generally based on themes of stalking and concealment, games like hide and seek, kick the can, the ghost in the graveyard."

Jeffrey had the capacity to hyperfocus. In elementary school he was a shy fearful boy. He performed poorly at school.

As an adolescent he would often walk around aimlessly. He would take up some activity, but would then lose motivation and drop it. He had an adolescent obsession with bones. He would collect killed animals from the road. He would "strip the flesh from the bodies of these putrescent road kills and even mount a dog's head on a stake" (Dahlmer, 1995). This has echoes of what the boys did in William Golding's *Lord of the Flies*.

When Jeffrey went to college, an experience that was unsuccessful, he took "a snake's skin with him". He performed poorly at College and soon dropped out. He "refused counselling. He had refused to get a job." Then he joined the army. The structure in the army certainly did help for a while. Certainly his alcoholism expanded in the army. After leaving the army, he deteriorated physically. He brought home "a dead raccoon in a gutter" and experimented on it. This has echoes of experimental murder (Dahlmer, 1995).

He suffered a good deal of depression. He was always a loner and shy. He always had major social interactional difficulties from early childhood. He was rather paranoid. He was in his own world, and had his own interests from childhood separate from other children. He was regarded as odd, intelligent and eccentric. He had no interest in group games (Masters, 1993).

Problems with Social Interaction

Jeffrey had major problems with social interaction. He was a very isolated child who was regarded as odd and eccentric. He walked up and down the school playground and did not socialise with other children.

Because of his identity diffusion, there was a great sense of emptiness inside. He lacked a cohesive sense of self. He wanted relationships, but in the Criminal Autistic Psychopathy way was unable to manage them and lacked the social know-how.

Persons with Criminal Autistic Psychopathy and serial killers are generally outsiders. They are alienated and detached from society. They cannot link in a close intimate way with human beings. They have a sense of deadness inside.

Masters (1993) stated that Jeffrey was very poor at "cocktail chat". He was very anti-authority and oppositional. He was naïve, immature, and lacked social cop-on.

Jeffrey was also a frotteur which means having sexual fantasies and rubbing against a non-consenting person. He stole a mannequin and used it as if it was a real body for sexual purposes. People were dehumanised in his vision. They were objects to be used as he wished. He operated on a part object relationships. Initially he began to drug his male companions and then used their bodies in this drugged state for sexual purposes. He would put his ear to their bodies listening to their hearts. He would engage in masturbation caressing of the body that was drugged.

He was repetitive in his activities and had preservation of sameness for example sitting in the same place at a bar every time. He had a confused androgynous sexual identity. This is typical of Criminal Autistic Psychopathy. He moved from drugged bodies to corpses. He went to a graveyard to get a corpse but the ground was too hard and he was unable to get it out (Masters, 1993). This all reflects his problems with normal social relationships.

In a way he was a kind of man disconnected from people on the planet. He was like a man floating in outer space. Because he was disconnected from the world and had no value on people, he was therefore dangerous and of course he simply used people as objects to gratify himself. In the therapeutic situation he was resistant, a very poor communicator, spoke very little. This is typical of persons with Autistic Psychopathy. It was impossible for therapists to make emotional contact with him. He would, also like Ludwig Wittgenstein did when dealing with the Vienna Circle, turn his back on people, in his case the therapists. Ludwig Wittgenstein was a philosopher who had Asperger's Syndrome (Fitzgerald, 2004). He showed rather paranoid ideas. Schizoid Personality Disorder is a diagnosis that is not uncommonly made in this situation as an alternative to Autistic Psychopathy. He came to relate in a kind of ritualistic way but these were empty interactions. He could occasionally tell lies.

Later in life he killed people so that he could lie down with them. It was a way of making social contact. According to his father:

> "in general, Jeff had simply wanted to keep people permanently, to hold them fixedly within his grasp. He had wanted to make them literally a part of him, a permanent part, utterly inseparable from himself. It was a mania that had begun with fantasies of unmoving bodies, and proceeded to his practice of drugging men in bathhouses, then on to murder, and finally, to cannibalism, by which practice Jeff had hoped to ensure that his victims would never leave him, they would be part of him for ever. He was socially awkward and was a lonely child.

His father describes Jeffrey's "emotions shaved down to a bare minimum". (Dahlmer, 1995).

This is a kind of definition of a person with Asperger's Syndrome a kind of pared down personality - a kind of shaved down personality.

Language

His father said he had a "monotonous" voice, which is typical of Autistic Psychopathy. He was excessively brief in his answers to questions. He had semantic pragmatic difficulties. He had problems initiating and sustaining conversations.

Jeffrey did not have schizophrenia as some suggested at his trial. He had odd ideas, but odd ideas are very common in persons with Autistic Psychopathy. Indeed delusional ideas, much less severe than schizophrenia, can occur in persons with Autistic Psychopathy.

Non-Verbal Behaviour

In adolescence:

"the loose-limbed boy disappeared, and was replaced by a strangely rigid and inflexible figure. He looked continually tense, his body weight very straight. When he walked his legs appeared to lock at the knees. This caused his legs to stiffen so much that his feet seemed to scrape across the ground, as if he were dragging them along rather than being carried by them."

He had an awkward walk. There were reduced non-verbal expressions in him (Dahlmer, 1995). He was charged with exhibitionism. Father also noticed a "deadness and emotional flatness" on his sons face (Dahlmer, 1995).

Some people thought he had charm, however, autistic charm is not uncommon. On balance he had very little of this.

Control and Narrow Interests

He liked the power and control that bomb making gave him. The movies that Jeffrey had watched included Blade Runner, Exorcist III, and other pornographic movies. Later he became interested in Anton la Vey's Satanic Bible. (Dahlmer, 1995) Persons with Autistic Psychopathy do have an interest in this kind of material. He had a tape recording of "numerology and the Divine Triangle" (Masters, 1993).

Jeffrey himself said "am I just an extremely evil person or is it some sort of satanic influence, or what?" (Masters, 1993). Jeffrey had also experimented with a séance trying to make contact with the dead (Dahlmer, 1995). He was into the occult and Satanism as persons with Autistic Psychopathy sometimes are. He was a compulsive masturbator.

Jeffrey wanted total control of the bodies of those that he killed to do what he wanted to do with to cut up, to masturbate towards, etc.. He was particularly obsessed by the chests of men. The first man he killed was a hitchhiker who had his shirt off on the day he met him. He loved touching the bodies of his victims. He opened the bodies up to see what was inside. He was fascinated by the autopsy scenes in the videotape "Faces of Death" (Dahlmer, 1995). He watched the Return of the Jedi repeatedly. Repetitive watching of videos is common in persons with Autistic Psychopathy. He was interested in making a shrine. He was fascinated with "the colours of peoples insides" (Masters, 1993).

Kelleher et al (1998) point out that Jeffrey Dahlmer wanted to manufacture "sex zombies" 'who would be forever at his command'"

Weak Central Coherence

Jeffrey's father said he himself was a man who "focussed on the minutiae of social life and often lost track of its overall design" (Dahlmer, 1995).

Identity

Jeffrey had identity diffusion and multiple selves. He was a Jekyll and Hyde character. His father said that in him he saw "a young man in whom something essential was missing" (Dahlmer, 1995). During a period of 24 hours he could be both a chocolate factory worker and a killer with multiple identities.

Criminal Activity

Earlier in his life, Jeffrey abused children and was imprisoned. His father asked the Judge not to let him out until he was treated. Personal rejection can precipitate killing, and this did happen in his case. He controlled people by drugging or killing them. He photographed bodies in various positions and this was part of his killing ritual. This was another way of holding on to them. Jeffrey "had not been able to reach orgasm unless his partner was unconscious" (Dahlmer, 1993).

Jeffrey also attempted a rather crude lobotomising of men. He would drug his victims with alcohol and sleeping tablets. It was noticed many times that the bodies would begin to smell and others would comment on this. He always had some excuse for the smell. Sometimes he was able to continue his relationship with the dead person through the skull in that he would keep this was again a part object. The skull was the symbol of the person. It was the symbol of the whole person. He used Baileys Irish Cream as part of the cocktail to drug people.

Jeffery seemed to want to merge with people in the bathhouses by drugging people and in that way he could in a way psychologically merge with them. Unfortunately of course they did then regain consciousness and could therefore leave him. To deal with this he killed at a later date.

According to Masters (1993):

"Jeffrey Dahlmer took a shower while there were two dead bodies in the bathtub, and he was sane. He drilled holes in the heads of living people to make them his unresisting companions, and he was sane. He ate a bicep that he had fried in a skillet, tenderised and sprinkled with sauce, and he was sane. For hours he lay with corpses, hugging them, cherishing them, and he was sane. He kept 11 assorted heads and skulls, and two complete skeletons, for eventual use in a homemade temple, and he was sane."

He suffered from a kind of existential meaningless.

Jeffrey's first murder occurred in 1978 and it was nine years before his next murder. He was a homosexual. He was noted to be very controlling. One man he killed he had no memory of doing the killing, and woke up in the morning with the man dead. It is difficult to fully explain this, but of course he was intoxicated himself. In terms of the killings, he always gave truthful and gave accurate reports. Murdering then became compulsive and he became addicted to it. He was unable to resist killing.

On one occasion he cut off the genitals of a man and placed them in his locker at work. He took photos of the dead bodies in various positions. It is hardly surprising he responded very poorly to group therapy after he was charged with the sexual assault. One person that he killed was "deaf and dumb" (Masters, 1993).

He would open up the bodies and "get an erection and lower himself onto the open body to have intercourse with the viscera, placing his penis literally within the body and ejaculating among its organs" (Masters, 1993). Clearly there was an absence of normal disgust and shame. This suggested abnormalities in the amygdala. He was into necrophilia.

He had to kill more frequently to try to get the same buzz. Like many serial killers he then became careless. Because of his difficulty of social relating and wanting to maintain contact it was then that he tried a form of leucotomy or lobotomy. He put a hole in the skull with a drill to attempt to do this.

Once Jeffrey had "thought of putting an electric wire through a hole in a live man's head and plugging the other end into the socket to see if an electric charge might keep him going" (Masters, 1993). The person was drugged at this stage while he was doing this. He was often suicidal throughout his life. He began to construct a shrine on a table. Certainly he said he felt no remorse at this point. He was handcuffing the man Edwards who was the last man he tried to kill ran out into the street and alerted the police which brought the whole business to an end. He was addicted to this kind of activity, felt completely driven, felt he could not control it and therefore his freewill was over come.

Dahlmer admitted everything and did not want this long drawn out court case. He was attracted by death and suicide. He hated thinking about his crimes. Nevertheless it is hardly surprising in prison he became more depressed and indeed suffered panic attacks. Nevertheless this changed mental state came after imprisonment not during the killing period. the idea that these people have zero anxiety is false.

Persons with Autistic Psychopathy experiment with human beings and are experimentalists. He was found guilty and given "over 900 years" (Masters, 1993). Another contradiction is that he may have had an element of the autistic superego because he acknowledged that "his acts were the worst imaginable and that there could be no forgiveness or salvation" (Masters, 1993).

For most people, Jeffrey Dahlmer equals evil. According to Stone (2005), "he commented that a biceps tasted like a steak". Bits of bodies were found all over his apartment.

During his adolescence he had fantasies of "rendering his victim unconscious and exposing their viscera". According to Simon (1996):

> "if he ate his victims, Dahlmer thought that they would provide him with strength and vitality, and they would live through him. So he treated a victims biceps and heart with a meat tenderiser, fried them in cooking oil, and added steak sauce."

Here he was literally merging or fusing with his victims.

At the end of his trial Jeffrey Dahlmer wrote "I knew I was sick or evil or both" (Masters, 1993). He appeared to glory in the publicity of the case as other serial killers have.

JOHN WAYNE GACY

Morrison and Goldberg (2004) stated that Gacy specialised in killing males and he killed 33. He engaged in sadistic sexual assaults, torture, and murder. Like a number of serial killers (e.g. Fred West) he buried them in his house. He got on very well with children and used to entertain them in a Children's Hospital. He was narcissistic, grandiose, and excellent at solving jigsaws. He was an autistic sensation seeker and showed autistic charm. He had identity diffusion with a multiple sense of self or selves. Gacy himself told Dr. Morrison "one body, two persons. The active person John Gacy has 15 characters, not personalities. Fifteen different characters evolved in one man. Sex drive, when it breaks in, its two people. John Gacy and Jack Hanley".

This has echoes of Jekyll and Hyde. This is identity diffusion or multiple selves of persons with Autistic Psychopathy. He described himself as a "motor mouth" He went on in monologues which are typical of persons with Autistic Psychopathy. He was rather paranoid about people. He had difficulty separating fact from fiction and differentiating males from females. He said he was "lonely and lost and confused" (Morrison and Goldberg, 2004). Maybe the killings were a pathological attempt to create a cohesive sense of self.

John Wayne Gacy "placed his mother's panties in a paper bag and hid them under his porch, often taking them out and caressing them" He was also very much into voyeurism with a telescope. He probably murdered eight women and in all these cases "the murder or attack was sadistic, sexual, violent, including incidents of stabbing, drowning, strangulation, mutilation, biting and or necrophilia" (Morrison and Goldberg, 2004).

He was excited by physical contact with dead bodies. Morrison and Goldberg point out that the "serial murderer is never as organised as a psychopath in his methodology" But a person with Autistic Psychopathy is different. Gacy showed autistic novelty seeking when he went to a mortuary, went into a coffin, and aroused himself. He had autistic charisma and charm. The police are unbelieving when they hear what serial killers have done. John Wayne Gacy used to play the clown in children's hospitals. He also "raped, tortured, and then buried many of his victims under the floorboards of his house" (Morrison and Goldberg, 2004).

He was paranoid and engaged in monologues rather than reciprocal social conversation. He had poor reality testing and a poor ability to separate fact from fiction. He had confused thinking and tried unsuccessfully to create a cohesive sense of self through killing. He was bewildered by the complexity of the social environment and was impulsive. Despite his contempt for people and his grandiosity he had low self-esteem. Even though he was intelligent he was regarded as being odd and worthless by his father who often told him so. He had Criminal Autistic Psychopathy. He had huge social interactional difficulties and merged with people. He showed weak central coherence with a great interest in detail. He was interested in aspects of mathematics. Murphy in *My Journey into the Mind of the Serial Killer*, *Irish Independent*, 3rd June 2004, stated that John Wayne Gacy may have buried some of his victims alive and that they then "desperately tried to dig themselves out" He poured lime over his victims who were buried under his home to "stifle the rotting stench, passing it off as dead mice to his wife" It is not that serial killers have no motive the excitement of killing is the motive. He blamed other people and for his problems for example blamed the government for executing him.

KARL PANZRAM

Karl Panzram once said: "I have no desire whatever to reform myself. My only desire is to reform people who try to reform me. As I believe that the only way to reform people is to kill 'em." (Gaddis & Long, 1970).
Karl also said "might makes right" (Gaddis & Long, 1970). He also said:

> "In my life time I have murdered 21 human beings, I have committed thousands of burglaries, robberies, larcenies, arsons, and last but not least I have committed sodomy on more than 1000 male human beings. For all these things I am not the least bit sorry. I have no conscience so that does not worry me. I don't believe in man, God, or Devil. I hate the whole damned human race including myself" (Gaddis and Long, 1970).

The famous psychoanalyst Karl Menninger wrote that Karl Panzram told him he would kill him if his chains were removed. He told Karl Menninger about his wish to better "the world in spite of his feeling that nearly all human beings were so bad that it would be better if they were all killed" (Gaddis & Long, 1970). He told Karl Menninger about "the incurable evilness of mankind, justifying complete extinction, including himself" (Gaddis & Long, 1970).
Karl Panzram murdered 21 people, had a major career in theft and was hypersexual with men. He had a disturbed delinquent childhood. He was also an arsonist. Homosexual abuse was often followed then by killing. He was full of anger and hatred towards human beings. He wanted to poison a whole city, he wrote his autobiography. He was very controlling and it was hardly surprising that he was hanged at the end when caught.

Personal History

Karl was born on the 28th of June 1891. He said, "I have been a human animal ever since I was born. When I was very young at 5 or 6 years of age I was a thief and a liar. The older I got the meaner I got" (Gaddis & Long, 1970). He was savagely beaten from childhood and indeed for much of the rest of his life. He had Oppositional Defiant Disorder and was extremely provocative. Nevertheless there was quite an intellectual aspect to him and despite a poor education he read works of philosophy. This would not be uncommon in persons with Autistic Psychopathy and reasonable intelligence. He was an autodictat.

The whippings in the reformatory school were extraordinary savage. The teachers would vie with each other to develop more savage methods of punishment. Clearly because of his Oppositional Defiant Disorder and Conduct Disorder he provoked endless punishments himself. He got back at some of the people in the school when he worked in the kitchen by urinating in their food. He attempted to poison a member of staff with rat poison. He was engaged in arson at that school and many other times during his life. He was very oppositional and stubborn and did not give in. Some of the beatings that he got were so savage that it is hard to believe he did not suffer some brain damage.

Karl's father had a bad temper and his mother was very rigid. His father had poor life management skills and was very restless. He drank excessively. He suffered from depression. Karl suffered from a good deal of illness in childhood, whether these were infectious illnesses often associated with Criminal Autistic Psychopathy is unclear. The reformatories and many of the prisons he was in were basically run along punitive sadistic lines. The prisoners were there to be abused and were very often. Nevertheless he met a few enlightened governors along the way.

Features of Autistic Psychopathy

Karl was "a silent, strange-eyed man" (Gaddis & Long, 1970). In prison, he was noted to be a "strange prisoner" (who) 'glowered, talked to himself, and grew angrier" (Gaddis & Long, 1970). He challenged authority at every possible opportunity. As a child he showed a lack of capacity to learn from experience or to manage his social relationships in a better way. He showed gross lack of empathy throughout his life. The vast majority of people he came into contact with he dehumanised and saw as objects. He was very much a loner. His philosophic autodictatic reading matter included Kant, Nietzsche, and Schopenhauer.

He began his first incarceration when he was 11 years. There is some evidence of an autistic narrative. He wrote, "What I have done to you, many others also do to you. Thus, we do each other as we are done by". He had Criminal Autistic Psychopathy but there were also massive environmental inputs. If there is a word called evil then it would apply to him.

Sodomy, Murder and Other Criminality

Karl engaged in sodomy with who ever he met whenever he felt like it. He said, "I knew more about sodomy than old boy Oscar Wilde ever thought of knowing" (Gaddis & Long, 1970).

He also wrote "I preyed upon the weak, the harmless and the unsuspecting". (Leyton, 1989).

When he worked with the Sinclair Oil Company he burnt down an oil well. He stole and bought a yacht and used it for killing. He worked in West Africa and on one occasion shot six men on a canoe and fed them to the crocodiles. He killed as young as 12 year olds whom he had sexually abused (Gaddis & Long, 1970). He also tried to murder when he was in prison and indeed did manage to murder one of the staff for which he was later hanged. He was full of hate, revenge, vengeance, and aggression. He had planned to blow up a train to kill people but didn't actually get to do it. He wanted to kill "millions of people" (Gaddis & Long, 1970). He wanted to start a war between England and America.

Earlier in his life, Karl told people about his killing activities but they did not believe him. He described how he had "raped a boy and strangled him with his own belt. He had bellowed that he would kill everybody down there and that he enjoyed killing people" (Gaddis & Long, 1970).

Killing was also a kind of enjoyable hobby for Karl. Nevertheless he was a good observer of the prison system. He wrote "in my life time I have broken every law that was ever made by both man and god. If either had made any more, I should very cheerfully have broken them also" (Gaddis & Long, 1970).

Like many persons of this type, he refused to be defended in court and said he would defend himself. He was incredibly fearful of seeing psychiatrists, or being described as insane. This is a very common fear of persons with Criminal Autistic Psychopathy. Being described as insane would be the ultimate insult. He wanted to be found guilty, he wanted to control everything, and he wanted to be hanged. In court he said "while you were trying me here, I was trying all of you too. I've found you guilty. Some of you I have executed. If I live, I will execute some more of you. I hate the whole human race" (Gaddis & Long, 1970).

In prison he was very much interested in the library books and particularly philosophy books. He wrote, "I hope they all go out like the Kilkenny cats did " (Gaddis & Long, 1970). He found the time waiting to be hanged very tedious. If they would not hang him he would kill himself. Indeed he did make one suicide attempt when it appeared as if they were not going to hang him. He did at one time fantasised about living on a deserted island with coconut trees. He hoped that he would and believed he would find peace in death. The night before he was hanged he sang a "pornographic little song" (Gaddis & Long, 1970).

Karl also wrote "if the law won't kill me, I shall kill myself. I fully realise that I am not fit to live among people in a civilised community. I have no desire to do so". Here he was being very controlling and dominating and requesting execution. As like Gilles de Rais, he was totally against the idea of reform.

Finally, he wrote, "with my last breath I intend to curse the world and all mankind. I intend to spit in the warden's eye or whoever places the rope around my neck when I am standing on the scaffold ... that will be all the thanks they'll get from me." (Gaddis & Long, 1970).

PETER KURTEN

Introduction

Peter Kurten was known as the Vampire of Dusseldorf (Lucas, 2002). He was a very famous German serial killer and spent almost half his life in prison where he had poor relationships with other prisoners.

Background

Peter's father was very harsh on him, abused alcohol, and was narcissistic and grandiose. His father was also imprisoned for sexual abuse. Peter ran away from home as a child but was caught. He claims a woman sexually abused him. He described himself as having "strong sexual passions" (Seaton Wagner, 1932).

Peter was rather an immature looking person and had an immature personality. He was "aloof and superior" to other people. He was of good intelligence. He first killed two boys when he was aged nine by drowning them (Lucas, 1974).

Kurten said, "I actually did have intercourse with female animals" (Berg, 1938). Kurten's sadistic tendencies are revealed quite early in his childhood in his love and enjoyment of the spectacle of animal slaughter. He claims to have first experienced lust under such circumstances". On one occasion "he seized a sleeping swan on the lake-side, cut off its head, and drank the blood" (Seaton Wagner, 1932). He described that when he was 13 years of age he "secured a complete orgasm by wounding. I attempted sexual intercourse with a sheep; whether it succeeded or the sheep would not keep still, I forget. I stabbed the sheep and at that moment ejaculated. I repeated that frequently for two or three years" (Berg, 1938).

Kurten was fascinated by fires, particularly ones that he ignited himself and would hang around as others started to put out the fire. This gave him enormous satisfaction. He set as a minimum 40 fires.

Many described him as a nice man. He also had a "Herostratism" according to Seaton Wagner (1932). He read a great deal and was very interested in the story of "Jack the Ripper" He tried to strangle a girl when he was 16 years of age. He was fascinated by the wax works museum where they showed serial killers. These were basically chambers of horrors (Seaton Wagner, 1932) and he would repeatedly visit these. In the waxworks museum, when he stood in front of the wax murderers he said "I am going to be somebody famous like these men one of these days!" (Seaton Wagner, 1932). He had problems relating to girls socially.

At the age of 19, Kurten attempted to gain sexual control over a former school fellow by terrorising her. "He threw an axe through the kitchen window, and the following day a heavy stone through the bedroom window. Five days later he fired five revolver shots at the girl's father, and two days later shot through the window of her parent's home, and wrote the girl a letter threatening her life if she did not give him a hearing" (Seaton Wagner, 1932).

Kurten took "advantage of every chance to enlarge his general education; and he had certainly come to amazing depths of knowledge of human nature and adjustment to environment. The foundation for this is to be found in his good memory". (Seaton Wagner, 1932). He had a massive memory for detail (Berg, 1938). He had threatened to kill his future wife if she did not marry him. "Yet, save for his wife, he had no human being who was dear to him, no friend, no comrade. His fellow workers considered him vain" (Berg, 1938). He dressed extremely well (Berg, 1938). He hit his wife only once. Nevertheless despite everything he was somewhat dependent on his wife and she was a kind of anchor for him in life. At the end, he was pleased that his wife got money given as a reward for information on him. Harold Shipman the serial killer expressed the same idea before he completed suicide about his wife.

Profile

Kurten was good with children as an adult. During the day he was a steady workman in a factory and during the night he was "a vampire prowling the woods and the lonely roads" (Seaton Wagner, 1932). He was a careful dresser and parted his hair very carefully. He was a great reader particularly of stories about killers and had, it appears a very high IQ. He was rather secretive a loner and had no intimate friends. He had a history of imprisonment and a great deal of burglary (Seaton Wagner, 1932).

In photographs he looked like a well dressed businessman. He was perverse and sadistic. He tormented animals as a child. Professor Berg a psychiatric expert told the court that "sadists are often very soft, gentle people" (Seaton Wagner, 1932).

Kurten had a tremendous autistic imagination. He was a cold, brutal, ruthless, cowardly killer. The psychiatric assessments which were carried out at the time were superb and equivalent to the best done today.

Peter Kurten was very much a Jekyll and Hyde figure. He seemed to be leading an ordinary life at one level and then at another level was involved in serial killing.

He confused fact and fiction. He had no remorse and suffered no guilt for his killings. He was a liar. He was fascinated by his killing activities as many serial killers are. Serial killers tend to be fascinated by the killings as facts that have taken place or events that have taken place. They often think about them without feeling or remorse. Peter excused his killing by the way he was treated in his previous life and also in prison. His story was that he was revenging himself on the human race. This is not untypical of a number of serial killers.

He adored the public discussions of his activities and the public reports in the newspapers of his trial. This gave him enormous narcissistic satisfaction.

Peter Kurten was a serial killer. In terms of his conscience, Peter Kurten said:

> "I have none. Never have I felt any misgiving in my soul; never did I think to myself that what I did was bad, even though human society condemns it. As I have figured it out, when I am executed, my blood and the blood of my victims will be on the heads of my torturers that is if there is such a thing as a Higher Justice. I have thought of the law of cause and affect, and on the law of the sufficient motive. There must be a Higher Being who gave in the first place the first vital spark to life. That Higher Being would also deem my actions good since I revenged injustice. The punishments I have suffered have destroyed all my feelings as a human being. That is why I had no pity for my victims" (Berg, 1938).

A judge once described him as being "the king of sexual delinquents" (Seaton Wagner, 1932). Peter said himself "I really always was in the frame of mind when I had the desire – or perhaps you could call it the urge – to kill somebody. The more people the better. Yes, if I had had the means of doing so, I would have killed whole masses of people. Every evening when my wife was at work I went prowling about for a victim" (Seaton Wagner, 1932). He also wrote that "the sex urge was always strong in me, particularly during the last years. But it was increased by the deeds in themselves. That was why I had to go the pit again and again to look for another victim" (Seaton Wagner, 1932). This shows the classical escalation of killing that takes place. Clearly fantasy played an incredibly important part leading up to the killings. When he was in prison he would "spend his spare time . . devising an entirely new set of crimes to avenge himself upon his oppressors when he came out" (Seaton Wagner, 1932).

This attack on the human race has echoes of Karl Prizam. His addiction to killing was evident by the fact that even when in prison he continued to kill, poisoning a couple of prisoners. This is also similar to other serial killers who have managed to kill in prison. Graham Young in Broadmoor did the same. He was also described as a werwolf and vampire because he would "receive the stream of blood that gushed from his victims wounds into his mouth" (Seaton Wagner, 1932).

Kurten was addicted to killing. The addiction worsened as he got older. He killed both children and adults. The killings were brutal, stabbing, and killing with a hammer etc. On one occasion, he sent a map to show where a body was buried to the police. He had autistic charisma and was considered attractive by women.

He said that "sometimes even when I seized my victims throat, I had an orgasm; sometimes not, but then the orgasm came as I stabbed the victim. It was not my intention to get satisfaction by normal sexual intercourse, but by killing. When the victims struggled she merely stimulated my lust" He was totally obsessed with finding potential victims and would prowl for hours on end, even on freezing cold nights (Berg, 1938).

Kurten said that when he tried "to kill a man with blows on the head with an axe. All these things gave me sexual satisfaction". At times he would return over and over again to the scene of the crime to where the body was lying. He changed his method of murder in order to increase the novelty of the killings (Seaton Wagner, 1932).

He also said "I told you already that throttling in itself was a pleasure to me, even without any intention to kill" (Seaton Wagner, 1932). On another occasion, he describes throttling a girl and "how the blood spouted from her mouth and in that way got my ejaculation". Like the Marquis De Sade, he discusses getting "a climax of enjoyment when I imagined something horrible in my cell in the evenings" This was when he was in prison. He was very conscious of the officers hunting him and this gave him great pleasure as well. He said "the main thing with me was to see blood". He was also a paedophile. After being caught, he said that he preferred "death to pardon. Though prison is different today from what it was in earlier times I see the contempt on the faces of the prison officials and the other prisoners" (Seaton Wagner, 1932). He was impatient for his execution.

"All the various cruelties which Kurten practiced served only the single purpose of achieving an orgasm" (Seaton Wagner, 1932). As it has been remarked, the coitus was often merely a sham manoeuvre of Kurten's, but in some cases he did achieve coitus by violence, as he confessed and that was proved" (Berg, 1938). He was an organised killer planning his killings. For Kurten, his activities were "90% sadism, 10% sense of injustice" (Berg, 1938).

Capture and Trial

A number of people escaped from him and one woman was able to identify him. He slept well at night after his killing spree.

Kurten was meticulous in the detail he gave about his crimes as was Albert de Salvo. He said at the end of his trial that: "there arrives for every criminal that moment beyond which he cannot go. And I was in due course subject to this psychic collapse". He also emphasised that "I never tortured a victim" (Berg, 1938).

The examining magistrate described him as "a man who scarcely knew any moral restraints, yet demanded for himself every sort of respect, nor did he suffer contradiction or challenge to his will" (Berg, 1938). He was clearly egocentric, narcissistic, and self-opinionated. He was also a manipulator and a liar. He discussed the great joy he got when he inflicted a wound and the victim starts bleeding.

What was surprising about Peter Kurten that he killed both sexes and different age groups. He did not specialise in one sex or age group like many other serial killers (Lucas, 1974).

He told the judge to punish him at his trial. He refused to make any appeal against the death sentence, which was handed down to him.

He had his last meal twice before being guillotined. He liked it so much he wanted it twice. He also said that if he was let out he would kill again . He had Criminal Autistic Psychopathy.

MARQUIS DE SADE

The Marquis de Sade wrote "either kill me, or take me as I am because I'll be damned if I ever change". In real life, he was a sexual sadist. Krafft-Ebing (1965) used the 1836 word "sadism" which had its origins in France as a medical term. The Marquis de Sade wrote of himself as follows in 1781,

> "Yes I am a libertine that I admit. I have conceived everything that can be conceived in that area, but I have certainly not practiced everything that I have conceived and never shall. I am a libertine, but I am neither criminal nor a murderer, and since I am obliged to place my apology next to my justification."

Indeed, he was a criminal but he was not a murderer.

In reality, the Marquis de Sade was not a serial killer, and the reader may ask why is he in this book. He spent his life in the pre-killing phrase. In his writings, he wrote about murderous sadistic criminal psychopathic acts that he took massive pleasure in. Guilt and remorse were absent from his character and were regarded as a weakness. Coward (1993) described him as having a "libertine dementia" This is a diagnosis not in the International Classification of Diseases. Myra Bremner (1991) has a good description of de Sade "serial killer" imagination when she wrote that "the 2,500 victims of both sexes in *Juliette* are not consenting, mostly are under 16 and many are under eight. This catalogue of atrocities belongs to the torture chamber not the bedroom, rapes split children open, pregnant women are disembowelled, babies cut to shreds, children flayed alive, eyes gauged out, boys castrated, parents forced to eat their children".

De Sade, in his novel *Juliette,* wrote, "how many crimes are incited by my prick", Noirceuil cried out (a man similar to de Sade). "What atrocities I commit in order to make it lose its firm with a little passion! There is no object on earth, which I am not ready to sacrifice to it! It is a god for me, Juliette, let it also be yours… a dour despotic phallus; offer incense to this superb deity. I would like it to receive homage from the entire planet". This has echoes of the thoughts of serial killers.

According to Phillips (2005), in *Juliette* "Marianne, Juliette's lovely 7 year old daughter, has already been raped by the appalling Noirceul. Having committed numerous atrocities on children, including the sodomising and murder of his own son, Noirceul asks mother's permission to murder Marianne in turn". Certainly this is the world of the serial killer. Phillips also notes that de Sade writes "mother natures laws unambiguously state that the mighty (should) harm the feeble, since for what other purpose have their powers been invested in the mighty?"

The idea that the strong should prey on the weak is a nasty vicious Sadeian philosophy. It is possible that vulnerable people, with also developed sadistic tendencies could be influenced by his writings and this may have happened with the Moors Murderer in England. Smith (2000) points out that de Sade wrote "in a famous scene in The 120 days of Sodom, De Sade depicts Pope Pius XI holding a black mass and having sex with his depraved anti-heroine Juliette on the main alter in St. Peter's, surrounded by hundreds of masturbating monks" De Sade also wrote in the *120 days of Sodom* "after having sheared off the boys prick and balls, using a red hot iron he hollows out a cunt in the place formally occupied by his genitals; the iron makes the hole and cauterises simultaneously... he fucks the patients new orifice and strangles him with his hands upon discharging". This is serial killing even if it only takes place in fiction. In one of De Sade's novels, according to Phillips (2005) "the man-hating Clairwil cuts off and embalms a monk's penis for use as a dido".

Coward (1991) points out that "The *120 days of Sodom* surely one of the most gruesome books ever written, is an account of a four-month orgy in a gothic castle where the reader is taken inexorably through a menu of 600 debauches" Coward also points out that there was "coprophilia, necrophilia, and torture of the most appalling forms of murder. There is no leer in De Sade's tone, no excitement, nothing remotely human, merely a cold, compulsive, efficient urge to catalogue".

De Sade in his book *Aline et Valcour* points out that "the good die by the hand of the wicked; the wicked die when they weaken; the merely reasonable are shown to lack human warmth; and the sensitive succumb to their inadequacies" These are issues of master slave relationships and really of Nietzsche's Superman.

For de Sade "all that counts is the continuation of life by procreation". This has a very modern 21st century ring about it in that reproducing genes is the critical tasks for human beings. Coward (1991) also points out that for de Sade "murder, war, and violent death in all its forms serve natures ends since they accelerate the release of re-usable matter. Conventional morality is unnatural since helping the weak to survive merely delays the process". He anticipated Freud and Hitler in different ways.

Coward (1991) points out that "de Sade's moral Darwinism allowed the fittest to survive on a diet of theft, murder, rape, and tyranny". Coward also says that "the Sadeian anti-hero exists in isolation in a world bereft of all feelings". He also points out that "de Sade dismisses established values as illusions, and insists, more blatantly than Freud ever dared and that sex rules the world and that there is no sex without cruelty". For de Sade, Coward (1991) points out that "cruelty as the necessary standard of private behaviour ... he is a terrorist of the psyche".

Hansford Johnson (1967) quoted de Sade "in a word, murder is a horror, but a horror often necessary, never criminal, and essential to tolerate in a republic".

Real serial killers prey on the weak and vulnerable and are contemptuous of other human beings. They lack, or have very little empathy for other human beings. Human beings are purely there for their pleasure, for satisfying their desires for abuse. Sade was narrowly focussed on sex like Sigmund Freud, but in a very different way. Nevertheless, the Marquis did sublimate his wish to be a serial killer in his imaginative writings. Freudian psychiatrists explain Sade as a man with problems with his Oedipus complex or unconscious conflicts. This is simplistic and grossly reductionistic, and not helpful.

De Sade spent about 30% of his life in either prison or psychiatric establishments. He was according to Davenport-Hines (2001) imprisoned for requesting of a "fan maker to whip him while he masturbated using a crucifix" Davenport-Hines (2001) states that that in 1772 he was "accused of sodomy and of poisoning two prostitutes to whom he had administered "candied lozenges" steeped in Spanish fly". Phillips (2005) notes, in relation to this, that when he was condemned to death for buggering and poisoning in actual fact he had been using Spanish fly, which is a well known aphrodisiac, which "also causes flatulence – an effect de Marquis found sexually arousing".

According to du Plessix Gray (1999), de Sade took perverse pleasure from "inhaling prostitutes farts". and stated that he was "a professor emeritus of crime" He made precise detailed records of his activities and indeed mathematical numbers were very important to him. Phillips noted that de Sade "recorded a number of his anal masturbations which mounted to 6,536 in the space of only 2½ years" Persons with Criminal Autistic Psychopathy are very interested in mathematics and making records of their activities.

Personal and Family History

According to Schaeffer (1999), de Sade's mother was a rather distant glacial figure who ended up her life in a convent. His father was rather naïve and tactless like himself and had poor life skills. His father abused his occupation and family position and lost a great deal and was described as persons with Autistic Psychopathy or traits often are by du Plessix Gray (1999) as "enigmatic".

According to Schaeffer (1999), as a child de Sade was "tyrannical and autocratic". He showed poor school progress even though he was very intelligent. He was a loner at school and always showed a poor capacity for reciprocal social relationships. He was a very immature and naïve child. He lacked common sense or social cop-on. He lacked "social know-how". He read a vast amount as a child and had a photographic memory.

Clare (1999) points out that by the age of four "… De Sade was a proud, obstinate, and physically aggressive boy, hypersensitive to insults, tyrannical, autocratic . . angry loner". Clare is correct when he wrote that it was not "at all easy to decide what kind of mental disorder his was". At that time Autistic Psychopathy was not well known to adult psychiatrists. Clare points out that "as he grew older, he constantly misjudged his impact on those around him" (Clare, 1999). This is typical of Autistic Psychopathy. Clare notes that de Sade was impulsive and obsessional, features that are very common in Autistic Psychopathy. Clare points out that this can be seen "not merely in the minute details of his sexual writings but in counting, checking, hoarding – all behaviours reflecting a remorseless drive to exercise control over the most intimate aspects of his life".

De Sade was always rather paranoid and hypersensitive to criticism. He had problems separating his imagination from external reality but nevertheless could be a good observer. His "best friends" were his books. He had no real friends in school. He was extremely egocentric, narcissistic, and grandiose. He thought of himself as omnipotent and wanted to be a god superior to everyone else – to have a life with no limits, no laws except his desire and the rules of the world should be made to suit him.

De Sade spent his life on a voyage of self-destruction like his father. He showed his naivety and tactlessness by continually exhibiting his perverse behaviour to an intolerant public who locked him up. He was like a man "from mars". He was an "alien" on planet earth. He was in a manner of writing in this world, but not of it and was in a way a lonely person. He approaches his perversions in a very organised way with meticulous attention to detail.

Du Plessix Gray (1999) noted that de Sade went to a Jesuit School and these schools put emphasis on "corporal punishment (and) sodomy". Nevertheless most ex-Jesuit boys did not became like de Sade. He was Jesuitical in his thinking. Gray (1999) also points out that in the army he was described as "deranged, but extremely courageous". Gray also states that he was "a misfit everywhere within his lifetime, a pariah even within his own cast" De Sade was an incredible sensation seeking or novelty seeker. He also showed evidence of Attention Deficit Hyperactivity Disorder hyperactive type, which can go with sensation seeking behaviour. He was very impulsive as well.

De Sade had a rather scientific and mathematical outlook and was a materialist. He rejected religion and other superstitions. He had sexual identity diffusion and was described by Phillips (2005) as a "rather effeminate-looking young man" He had identity diffusion. Women found him attractive and he showed an autistic charisma. He blamed nature (biology) for his behaviour and was very advanced at that time giving so much weight to nature, which at a later date was defined in genetic terms. He suggested that you could not change his nature and therefore he did not wish and could not be cured. He was correct about this. The same might be said of many serial killers although criminal behaviour in general does tend to 'burn-out' in the latter stages of life.

De Sade – Literature, Philosophy, and Drama

According to Coward (1991), he was an "elusive subject" He was totally subversive of contemporary values. Coward points out that for "Sainte Beuve the two presiding geniuses of romanticism were in order, Byron and de Sade".

De Sade was quite Byronic in certainly some of his activities particularly his sexual activities. He went further than Byron (Fitzgerald, 2001). Coward also states that "for Baudelaire, he was the flower of evil, and Flaubert loved his dirty talk. Swinburn was fascinated".

Byron was also interested in his work. Byron who indulged in incest and promiscuity was not too far removed in behaviour from de Sade. Leith (1991) states that for years "literary Sadists such as Roland Barthes accused critics of avoiding de Sade for fear of seeming politically incorrect". Hitchings (1999) points out that for writers "like Ronald Barthes and Octavio Paz, Angela Carter, and Simone de Beauboir, de Sade's work is a departure, a springboard to diffuse musings on sex, morality, art, and the will". Thorne (2004) correctly out that de Sade was "the most shocking, outrageous and obscene novelist whoever lived".

Coward (2005) in a review of Phillips (2005), *How to Read de Sade,* that progressive spirits (from Baudelaire to the Surrealists and Postmodernist) have hailed him as the apostle of freedom, the ultimate taboo eater and the trail blazing transgressor of an over-regulated moral and social codes". He also points out that de Sade "helped to move western civilisation away from god centred creation to man-centred materialism". This was his only positive achievement but he did it in a totally unacceptable way.

Phillips (2005) points out that de Sade was a "creature of uncertainties and contradictions, but ultimately a profound and radical thinker, an author of considerable intellect and erudition". Phillips points out that Sade demonstrated "sadistic cruelty of certain scenes and the philosophical justifications for this cruelty".

De Sade's novels have "torture and murder, they depict acts of paedophilia, sadomasochism, fetishism, and perversion. He was indeed a criminal. Phillips (2005) points out that de Sade "fearlessly explores the darker side of human nature... the objectification of human beings, the utter selfishness of lust, the tyranny of an ego unfettered by laws, or lacking the humanising influences of socialisation" There are no philosophical justifications for sexual abuse or perverse behaviour towards human beings unless one was a Nazi. Phillips says that "de Sade's obscene writings cannot be properly read outside this literary historical context" This is not so. His interests were not historically based but emerged from the core of his personality his Criminal Autistic Psychopathy.

De Sade's writings and behaviour were not then or now the norm for civilised behaviour. He shows an autistic narrative in that "the very mobility of de Sade's thought and the sometimes allusive character of meaning in his writings is intriguing and stimulating". His autistic narrative is shown in what Phillips describes as "Sade's textual games compelled the reader to play a more active part in the creative process through conjecture and speculation". This kind of writing is also seen in Ludwig Wittgenstein and Jacques Lacan and is due to their Semantic Pragmatic language problems.

De Sade's autistic narrative is at times not very clear, exceptionally condensed, and ignoring the reader's position. Schaeffer (1999) stated that he wrote "mad letters" which were disjointed. According to Phillips (2005), "the structuralist Ronald Barthes who completely divorced literature for reality, reading the scenarios of de Sade's fiction as safely distant from the moral questions that would arise, were they to take place in the real world" . Barthes makes no sense with this position and indeed this is an absurd position.

Du Plessix Gray (1999) quotes Goncourts when they wrote "in Flaubert there is truly an obsession with de Sade: he racks his brains to find sense in that madman". Flaubert had Asperger's Syndrome. For Baudelaire "to understand evil, one must always return to de Sade, that is, to natural man". The first prominent medical treatise that referred to de Sade was Krafft-Ebing's *Psychopathia Sexualise*. His novels cannot be seen as just texts. This is absurd. This is how Lacan would see them. The man and the text cannot be separated. He was an evil perverse sadomasochistic man who used and abused people for his own desires. Unfortunately, Bruno Bettelheim got sucked into his perversity. It is interesting that Bruno Bettelheim in his book *The Empty Fortress: Infantile Autism and the Birth of the Self*, makes reference to Marquis De Sade when he writes "some modern writers are beholden to this level of personality development as was Marquis De Sade, for example in a previous century. As he tried to act out his sexual fantasies in a world which therefore felt obliged to lock him up, so have mental patients always done" This is a very disturbing comment on de Sade from Bruno Bettelheim and Bettelheim shows a lack of appreciation of de Sade's cruelty.

The best work, I have read on de Sade was by Myra Bremner who was very critical and rightly so of the republication of *Juliette* by de Sade. She believed that the publishers should "rescind this recent publication of Juliette by De Sade or be prosecuted under the Obscene Publications Act 1959. Civilised society depends on competing freedoms being used reasonably – freedom to publish is no exception". Myra Bremner is a rare woman who calls "a spade a spade" and does not go along with the trendy French intellectuals and the French intelligencia who have raised de Sade's perverse writing to the level of French literary cannon. One must ask what are French standards? What is beyond the limits in France? Are these French philosophical justifications for paedophilia, perversion of every sort and child sadomasochism? Has French intellectual life lost its way?

If de Sade had not been locked up in prisons and mental hospital he would not have had the time to write all these perverse works and thousands of letters that he wrote endorsing his perverse values which antedated Nazi texts. His writings were very repetitive, not surprisingly given his narrow interests and his Criminal Autistic Psychopathy. Davenport-Hines points out that "de Sade's prison letters can seem interminable, monotonous, inexorable, they are as repetitive and as humorous as his novels" There were many people in France at the time who were engaged in perverse sexual practices but they hid them and did not flaunt them like de Sade.

Weightman (1992) points out that "the masochistic element was strong in de Sade himself and, like Proust's" Monsieur de Charles, he could not always find people to whip him convincingly enough, so perverse, alas, is human nature" He also makes a very important point that "in the amoral atmosphere of the time, Sade's behaviour might have passed unnoticed, but had he gone about it with discretion. But, being ungovernably obsessive and, besides, distinctly cracked in a lordly way, he fell foul of two different authorities". This is because of his tactlessness, lack of commonsense, and lack of empathy.

Persons with Criminal Autistic Psychopathy often come into contact with the police because of their lack of 'cop' on and discretion. He also points out that "given a few grains of commonsense and a less determined mother-in-law, he might have led a busy life as a closet sadist and flagellator, and have remained unknown". But persons with Criminal Autistic Psychopathy do not have commonsense. Weightman quotes Donald Thomas that the Marquis was "a barer of bad news about the human race". Donald Thomas's (1992) book was The Marquis De Sade. . De Sade had a very narrow singular focus. He was very much into control, into sadomasochism, into perversion. He wanted to transcend the world and be a god in his own way.

Phillips (2005) stated that de Sade rejected "the very notion of crime". He was the ultimate transgressor and the philosopher of paedophilia and sexual perversion. His interest in plays and dramatic works focussed on his narrow perverse interests where sexual perversion had the same moral value as any non-perverse behaviour.

LEE HARVEY OSWALD

Lee Harvey Oswald had poor life management skills and an erratic work record. He had identity diffusion. He defected to Russia and then came back to the United States again. He was a man with narrow ideas and narrow interests. He was obsessed with communism and Marxism. He was an intelligent person. He was a great reader and an autistic drifter. He was very narcissistic, grandiose, and was an angry secretive person. He was rather paranoid. He had a poor sense of self. He was angry at Kennedy's treatment of Cuba and Fidel Castro.

Oswald had Autistic Psychopathy. He was extremely controlling. He was a lonely man. He had little sense of humour. He was very intense about his special interest that is his hatred of America. He was a liar but also had an autistic superego. He could engage in monologues and could talk for a couple of hours non-stop at a time. He was very hard to get to know and an enigma and was interested in political ideas particularly Marxism. He was very naïve about Marxism. In some ways he was generally naïve. When he spoke to the journalist Johnson she thought that all his life "he had been all his life a machine, collaborating social justice" (Davison, 1983).

He was an outsider but wanted to be famous and had a huge opinion of himself. He possibly got his Autistic Psychopathy from his mother who was an unusual woman who for example buried her husband the same day that he died. Early on in his life, Oswald was interested in astronomy, liked animals, and history as persons with Autistic Psychopathy often do and was autodictatic. He dropped out of school. He was examined by a psychologist and found to have "a considerable amount of impoverishment in the social and emotional areas" (Davison, 1983). He had poor social relationships and spent a lot of time by himself. He had problems with social know-how and social cop-on and was naïve.

Oswald received a psychiatric diagnosis of "schizoid" (Davison, 1983). The Psychiatrist said there was "apparent in his extreme withdrawal and the depth to which he seemed to live in a fantasy" (Davison, 1983) He had a very poor capacity for empathy and was introverted. He had a confused identity. He was oppositional. He loved books particularly Encyclopaedias. A fellow student Edward Voebel said that "people just didn't interest him generally" because he was "living in his own world" (Davison, 1983). He confused fact from fiction.

> "Psychiatrist and author Edwin Weinstein believes that many potential assassins take up a political cause to give themselves a sense of identity. Several other American assassins have identified strongly with a political group – John Wilkes Booth with the Confederacy, Sirhan Siren with the Palestinians" (Davison, 1983).

A famous book the *Criminal Personality* by psychiatrist Samuel Yochelson and his associate psychologist Stanton Samenow noted that recidivist criminals were self-centred and secretive. They saw themselves as "unique". They were "chronically restless, dissatisfied, and angry" They were into novelty seeking and fantasy. They were rather narcissistic and grandiose. They were loners, egocentric and saw other people as there to be used. They tended to blame others. They searched for "power, control, and excitement" (Davison, 1983).

Oswald worked in radar during his time in the marines. He was court-martialled there for having non-army weapons. He defended himself, which is typical for persons with Asperger's syndrome. He had little capacity for "irony" (Davison, 1983). He read George Orwell's book *Animal Farm* in a concrete fashion (Davison, 1983). He had a sense of destiny for himself and his own greatness and uniqueness. He was a confused and contradictory person. He was a user of people.

Criminal Autistic Psychopaths like Oswald provide the greatest risks to senior political figures. He had a rigid personality type. He wrote at times in a rather autistic narrative style that was hard to follow. He lived in his own autistic world and did suffer from depression. He admired J. Edgar Hoover and Mao Tse-Tung both of whom had Asperger's syndrome. His political thinking was confusing and was in the confused autistic thinking style. He was motivated entirely by personal matters and there was no conspiracy.

RICHARD MACEK

Morrison *et al* (2004) in *My Life Among the Serial Killers* give an excellent description of Richard Macek. He had a clear identity diffusion and androgyny. He was "physically odd..with a peculiar combination of male and female characteristics" Identity diffusion or androgyny is often seen in Autistic Psychopathy. He was rather paranoid about people. He was very sensitive to frustration and rejection. He was sensitive to noise for example "the low voices outside the door, including one of the guards got under his skin". He disliked people looking at him. He had a very immature personality. Morrison *et al* points out that "it is not uncommon for serial killers in general to believe that things have the characteristics of people". Of course they often reduce people to the level of inanimate objects.

Persons with Autistic Psychopathy are often fascinated by textures and he would steal ladies undergarments and chew on them with his teeth to enormous satisfaction. John Gacy another serial killer with Criminal Autistic Psychopathy was also fascinated by the touch of women's undergarments.

Persons with Autistic Psychopathy often have problems with the concepts of time, past, present, and future. They can get stuck in the present time only. Morrison *et al* (2004) point out that Macek was very capable of "re-living his horrors as if they were happening in real life" He suffered like many people with Autistic Psychopathy from hypochondrical symptoms. He experienced a great emptiness in his psyche and in his sense of self. He showed his capacity for autistic narrative in that it was difficult to follow his letter writing, they did not communicate real feelings or give a clear sense of context and were made up of ordinary common phrases from general linguistic discourse that he had been exposed to, i.e. clichés. He showed evidence of semantic pragmatic language difficulties. He showed evidence of impulsivity and was very intelligent. He would make rather random answer to questions that did not make any sense. He spoke in an autistic monologue. He showed evidence of a semantic pragmatic language problem. He had a false self and could present a façade of normality.

Morrison *et al* (2004) wrote that Macek said "my skin just hanging on my bones". This shows that he was on the verge of psychic disintegration and identity diffusion. Surprisingly his family life appeared to the outsider as being normal. This again is the Jekyll and Hyde position. He spoke in monologues and had a rigid obsessional personality. He lacked the capacity at a deep psychological level for authentic interpersonal reciprocal social relationships. He played at relationships rather than feeling inside them. He showed his difficulty with reality testing with his tendency to merge with people. Persons with this condition often fuse with people and lose their ego boundaries. In this situation it seems he has combined two people into one. He was controlling and dominating as when he got the dentist to take out his teeth. Control is central to Criminal Autistic Psychopathy.

Richard Macek killed about eight people (Morrison and Goldberg, 2004). His killing was extremely perverse, sadistic, and included knifing victims, some victims were strangled. He was also a necrophiliac and bit his victims. He had Criminal Autistic Psychopathy. He was a serial killer of the female sex. He also showed further evidence of his problems with reality testing with his difficulty knowing whether a woman he had attacked was alive or dead. He terminated his own life by self-harm and so remained in control.

RICKY GREEN

Ricky Green was a classic serial killer who savagely attacked and lacerated the bodies of his victims. He was a perverse sexual sadist and mutilator of bodies. He showed no evidence of guilt, conscience, or remorse. He had huge difficulties with social interactional skills, had a piercing gaze and was hypersensitive to rejection, an experience which could trigger killing. There was an environmental element to his personality development in that he was abused as a child and there was much domestic violence in his family (Tancredi, 2005). Green was cruel to animals and had a history of arson attacks. It would appear that from childhood he had developed chronic Post Traumatic Stress Disorder. He was a Jekyll and Hyde figure. In the book of the same name, the Jekyll and Hyde figures had Autistic Psychopathy, as did its author R. L. Stevenson. The killing instinct in Ricky Green was uncontrollable. Tancredi felt that "the mirror-neuron system of Green's brain most likely imitated the behaviour of his father and siblings, including the way they handled anger, rage, and lack of control of their impulses and desires".

Tancredi also pointed out that Ricky Green probably also had "a relatively ineffective inhibitory system (limbic structures, anterior cingulate cortex, orbito frontal cortex), which he dampened further by alcohol consumption".

THOMAS WAINEWRIGHT

In some ways, Wainewright was Byronic in his behaviour. He was a liar and a strange enigmatic man. He had Criminal Autistic Psychopathy. He had a large head, suffered from identity diffusion, and showed multiple selves, no remorse. He liked animals. He was naïve and immature, artistic and a liar. Although his poisonings were not proven, the evidence is pretty strong against him and what strongly supports this is the multiple poisonings.

John Carey on the back of the book in the *Sunday Times* described him as a "ruthless murderer and an outstanding painter and critic". Edward White in the *Financial Times* described him as a "sociopath murderer". He was convicted of fraud and sent abroad on a convict ship to Van Diemen's Land. Oscar Wilde wrote in *Pen, Pencil, and Poison* "the fact of a man being a poisoner is nothing against his prose". His dates are 1794 – 1847. He was "an ingenuous and unscrupulous criminal" (Motion, 2000).

Waineright poisoned a number of people including his mother-in-law. These killings were for financial gain. This is not serial killing but multiple killing. He was an evil man but he was also a cultured man and a significant artist. He was Hyperkinetic and dressed as a dandy. He showed unemotional callousness. He confused fact and fiction. He was convicted for fraud. His mother was quite an intelligent well-educated woman and died when she was 21 years of age. His grandfather then reared him. He blamed his upbringing and other people for his problems. He lived beyond his means and did not have enough money to maintain his lifestyle. It was for this reason that he began to get people to take out insurance policies with him as the beneficiary and then to poison them. He was a rake. He read a great deal. There was no doubt he was a man of talent. He was an irresponsible gambler like Byron and had some similarities to Oscar Wilde.

Helen, his sister-in-law, was one of the girls he sent to take out an insurance policy and who was then poisoned by him. As far as it can be ascertained, he also poisoned his mother-in-law. It appears he used strychnine and also gave her antinomy. It is not detected at the post-mortem. The insurance companies refused to pay and court cases followed. At the end of the day, he was convicted of fraud and transferred to Van Diemen's Land as a convict and serving a life sentence. He suffered as well from depression. It is not absolutely clear how many he may have poisoned. He was naïve, impatient, and reckless in engaging in legal action. He was also impatient. He never admitted his guilt and always blamed others. He was harshly treated in Van Diemen's Land. It seems that his handling of the authorities there in the early stages were somewhat tactless which aggravated the situation. He abused opium. He was "one of the best Australian portrait painters of his day" He painted many in Hobart. He did a self-portrait called "The Head of a Convict". He liked animals.

Persons with Criminal Autistic Psychopathy often like animals and he was very good with his cat. Unfortunately he did not treat humans in the same way. Humans were simply there to be used as objects by him for financial gain. He was talented in art, but was savage in his killings. He was also described as "cold, vain, silly, penal, and heartless". He was a multiple killer who killed for profit. (Motion, 2000). He had Criminal Autistic Psychopathy.

GEORGE CHAPMAN

George Chapman's real name was Severin Klosowski and he was born on the 14th of December 1865 in Poland. He trained as a "barber/surgeon" (Adam, 1930) He was a rather restless Hyperkinetic individual. He moved jobs frequently. He showed poor life management. He appeared to be a bigamist and was also very promiscuous. He also went through a number of pretend marriages where he said he was getting married, went off with a woman, and returned and pretended to have gone through a marriage ceremony. He took the name Chapman from Annie Chapman, a woman that he had a relationship. Annie left him and was not killed. After she left, he called himself George Chapman.

He carried out a number of crimes which were described as showing "remarkable recklessness and daring, having for their primary purpose and idée fixe the pursuit, the capture, and the destruction of women" He formed a relationship with a Mrs. Spink who had a child who was grossly neglected by them both. Chapman bought a small "sailing and rowing boat" but was a very clumsy and hazardous sailor. Then Chapman bought some poison from a chemist and marked the bottle poison. Persons with Criminal Autistic Psychopathy are particularly interested in poisons. He gave this to Mrs. Spink in increasing doses and finally killed her. Chapman feigned grief when she died, but on the day she died he "opened his premises at the usual time".

The next woman he pretended to marry was Bessie Taylor. He was very "cruel to her, abusing her a good deal, and even going to far as to threaten her with a revolver". (Adams, 1930) Again he poisoned her and she gradually deteriorated and died. The next woman he killed was Maud Marsh, but her family became suspicious. She again began to develop a mysterious illness which people could not fathom. When her mother became very suspicious, he then gave her an increased dose and killed her. The poison was actually antimony. This was found at the post-mortem and the other women were then exhumed and it was also found on them. They found medical books that he had in his house. Sir Edward Carson, who prosecuted Oscar Wilde, prosecuted Chapman who was sentenced to death.

"Antimony, being colourless, odourless, practically tasteless, and easily soluble in water, is a very dangerous poison from a homicidal point of view". (Adams, 1930) This has echoes of Graham Young, the multiple killer who also used it. Chapman showed evidence of carelessness, even though he was an intelligent man, which led to him being caught. This recklessness increased as he got older and carried out more crimes but it may also be a way of increasing the excitement that comes with recklessness. His murders were for "gross personal gratification". When he was caught, he told lies but was easily caught out in these. He was a "braggart" and was egocentric and narcissistic. He was a bit of a Walter Mitty character and was similar in some ways to Don Quixote, a fictional character who had Asperger's Syndrome.

Chapman photographed the women whom he afterwards murdered. He was tactless and unempathic and when in his pub he expressed "pro-Boar sympathies" in London. He was fascinated by criminal matters and liked to associate with police officers. He had an extraordinary control over women who did not seem able to leave him despite his abuse of them. This domination and control can be seen in Criminal Autistic Psychopathy. Some people speculated that Chapman was Jack the Ripper who was operating in London at exactly the same time that Chapman was operating. I do not believe so. (Adam, 1930)

ANDREI ROMANOVICH CHIKATILO

Serial killing is a universal phenomenon. Andrei Romanovich Chikatilo was known as the Rostov Ripper. He was a married schoolteacher and was one the most savage brutal schoolteachers of all time. He was into sexual attacks, mutilation of bodies, cannibalism and torture. He killed children as well as adults.

He was called The Red Ripper and was 44 year of age. He killed and mutilated at least 12 victims. This is a phenomenon not uncommon in persons with Criminal Autistic Psychopathy who often leave their mark. He became sexually excited by the girls struggling before he killed them. He masturbated as he killed them and bit their bodies. His killing behaviour escalated, as he got older. (Morrison *et al*, 2004). He showed no evidence of conscience, remorse, or guilt. Chikatilo showed no evidence of psychosis at his trial and blamed others, which is common with serial killers.

He was an intelligent teacher and was shy. He had major reciprocal social interactional problems. Peter Conradi (1992) noted that at work he was described as a "human robot". This is a term sometimes applied to people with Criminal Autistic Psychopathy. Conradi also notes that in court he was described as a person who "demonstrated animal cruelty and ruthlessness as he cold-bloodedly knifed his victims, literally tearing apart live women and children". To compare him to an animal is to do injustice to many animals. In court, he was accused of 53 murders. He was a Jekyll and Hyde figure who chose vulnerable people to be his victims. He was very excited by their slow deaths. He was an organised serial killer. Sadistic killing was his method of getting sexual satisfaction.

BYKOV

"A less well-known brigand, Bykov, was the leader of a band in Siberia. Along with cruelty he displayed a degree of scientific curiosity unusual in one of his profession: he ordered one of his followers to disembowel a pregnant woman and explained at his trial that he wanted to see what position the foetus occupied in the womb" (Chalidze, 1977). This is experimental murder which is sometimes observed in Criminal Autistic Psychopathy.

ROBERT BERDELLA

Robert Berdella killed "to see what happened" (Morrison and Goldberg, 2004). He was experimental and was interested in the occult like many persons with Criminal Autistic Psychopathy. He kept a detailed diary of his activities. He tortured people in a meticulous way. Persons with Criminal Autistic Psychopathy often get on well with pets and this was Berdella's position. He was like Doctor Spock in Star Trek who shows clear evidence of Autistic Psychopathy. He had autistic interests. He also photographed his victims. He killed people slowly. He bit his victims. His victims were dehumanised objects for him. He kept meticulous documentation of his activities. He again was a Jekyll and Hyde figure. He was also a community activist like Harold Shipman. He died of natural causes while incarcerated.

MICHAEL LEE LOCKHART

Michael Lee Lockhart was a serial killer who kept meticulous records of his crimes. He showed poor self-care, which is not uncommon in persons with Criminal Autistic Psychopathy. He wanted to leave his mark on life and to be seen as a celebrity. Lockhart was egocentric, narcissistic, and grandiose. He felt drawn to kill. He was a Jekyll and Hyde figure who was somewhat of a loner. He was a novelty seeker and sensation seeker. He could show a pseudo-normal façade.

Morrison and Goldberg (2004) describe one murder where he sodomised a woman and "slashed at her with a knife until she was dead". He felt relaxed after a killing. He had an immature personality. He suffered from identity diffusion and a very uncertain sense of self. He was hypochondriacal. He could be diagnosed with Alexithymia which is often confused with Autistic Psychopathy (Fitzgerald *et al* (2006). Lockhart spoke with a kind of "verbal diarrhoea" He had Criminal Autistic Psychopathy.

SYLVESTRE MATUSCHKA

When Matuschka wrecked a train, he would pretend to be one of the victims of the train crash. He said when he was caught "I wreck trains because I like to see people die. I like to hear them scream. I like to see them suffer" (Lucas, 1974). The train crash was a sexual event for him that excited him. He was a courageous man in the 1st World War.

He was a rather Walter Mitty/Don Quixote character, fictional figures with Asperger's Syndrome like the writer Cervantes. He had great fantasies about solving the world's problems. Some of these were of great engineering projects. He suffered from identity diffusion and multiple selves which he labelled various Leos. He had the kind of delusions you sometimes see in Criminal Autistic Psychopathy, - autistic delusions. Lucas (1974) points out that he showed "a recurrent sadistic sexualisation of destructiveness" As usual he blamed others for what he did. He was certainly egocentric and grandiose. Matuschka himself stated that he acted under "some irresistible influence" (Lucas, 1974).

DENKE, GEORG GROSSMAN, AND FRITZ HAARMANN

Denke was a serial killer and a German organ-grinder. Denke had 12 bodies in a bag when caught, having cut them up. He kept a detailed diary of his killings (Seaton Wagner, 1932). He killed about 30 people in all. A smell emanated from his flat just like Jeffrey Dahlmer when he kept bodies there. When Denke was caught he completed suicide. He was a very solitary man.

Georg Grossman killed during the 1930s in Germany. He would meet people coming off the trains at railway stations, offer them accommodation and then strangle them. He would sell their clothes. He also sold "meat" from their bodies. He was described as "the most dreadful sexual-pathological murderer of all time" (Seaton Wagner, 1932).

Cawthorne (2002) stated that Fritz Haarmann was the "Butcher of Hanover" – "Werwolf of Hanover", "Vampire of Hanover". He probably killed over 50 people "by biting out their throats, and selling their flesh to unwitting customers on the black market that flourished in Germany following the end of World War One" He was also a child abuser who had negative upbringing. He sexually abused his victims. Like many of these serial killers, he did not want to be seen as crazy in any way or having a mental illness. He was beheaded. He had Criminal Autistic Psychopathy.

WILLIAM HEIRENS

William Heirens was a highly intelligent medical student. According to Lucas (1974), in 1946 he raped and murdered a six-year-old girl. He also raped and mutilated other adult women. Once he wrote on the wall after he killed a woman "for gods sake catch me before I kill again. I cannot control myself" (Lucas, 1974).

Heirens had been a thief for quite a long time before he started to murder. He was a transvestite and had sexual identity diffusion. He had poor social relationships and was a very shy person. He had Criminal Autistic Psychopathy. He had a history of sexual excitement from stealing women's undergarments and kept a large collection of these in his house. This is something common in Criminal Autistic Psychopathy. He had irresistible impulses. He suffered from identity diffusion, multiple selves and he claimed one of these selves carried out the crimes. These multiple selves are often seen in Criminal Autistic Psychopathy. Lucas points out that he was a "shy", "nervous" and "unsociable" individual. He was quite religious.

ALFRED CHARLES WHITEWAY

Alfred Charles Whiteway murdered and attacked the sexual organs of his victims (Lucas, 1974). He also sexually interfered with his victim after death. He was a moody individual who had a short temper. He was obsessed with knives and bodybuilding. He had spent time in a reformatory earlier in his life. He was a sadistic sex killer and had Criminal Autistic Psychopathy with no signs of guilt, remorse, or conscience (Lucas, 1974). He was a Jekyll and Hyde character with a false self, which fooled people, but he was also a vicious sadistic sexual killer. He had narrow interests, e.g. killing, bodybuilding and cycling. He suffered from identity diffusion and a disturbance of a sense of self.

PETER MANUEL

Peter Manuel was involved in serial killings, but there was no evidence of any "attempt at any kind of sexual assault". (Lucas, 1974). He was also a housebreaker. He was found guilty of seven murders. He was addicted to killing. He was a great reader and an autodictat and a visual artist as well as being musical. He was very controlling and dismissed his defence counsel during the trial. This is not uncommon behaviour by persons with Criminal Autistic Psychopathy. Before he was hung, he admitted to three other murders and when you add in the murdered taxi driver, his total comes to twelve. He made a confession and then withdrew it, which is not uncommon in Criminal Autistic Psychopathy. His killing was related to the thrill of the kill and not sex.

GORDON CUMMINGS

Gordon Cummings was a Walter Mitty type of serial killer with Criminal Autistic Psychopathy. His peers did not like him. He was a sadistic sexual killer, mutilating the bodies (Lucas, 1974). He had identity diffusion or multiple selves. He was regarded in London as a second ripper. Lucas (1974) described the killings as taking place during the 2nd World War and Cummings was hanged during an air raid.

BRUNO G

Haire (1952) describes Bruno G. a sexual murderer. Bruno G. was timid, lacked a spirit of gaiety as a child, and suffered from depression. He felt eyes were staring at him during the night and he had little sensitivity to pain. He spoke in a low voice. He was narcissistic. He described himself as "curious, taciturn, and credulous" but not easily accessible. He was fearless. He had a great imagination. He hated large groups and kept to himself. He was a compulsive masturbator. He was a fetishist. He was a voyeur. It appears that he had Criminal Autistic Psychopathy.

JOHN REGINALD CHRISTIE

10 Rillington Place was where John Reginald Christie lived. John Reginald Christie's was born on the 8th of April 1898. He came from a strict background. He was a good singer. He was interested in dead bodies and fascinated by them. He was into theft. He had a poor work record. He was somewhat of a fantasist. He had a deep hatred of women. The pleasure that he got from killing was unlike any other pleasure he had in his life before. It gave him an enormous sense of contentment and fulfilled his novelty seeking wishes. It then became a way of life. He mutilated these bodies. Another man was hanged for his activities. Christie confessed voluntarily. There was much planning in his activities. He was eventually hanged. (Cawthorne, 2002).

According to Martin Fido (2001), Christie gave "callous and jocular accounts of his monstrous actions" This can occur in Criminal Autistic Psychopathy. He not only strangled his victims, but also sexually assaulted at the same time and buried their remains in his garden. He had spent time as a special policeman and indeed had been a schoolmaster (Fido, 2001). His father was authoritarian, controlling, and a cold figure. Christie showed necrophiliac behaviour. He had sexual relations with unconscious bodies. He used to gas "his victims into a state of unconsciousness". He was described as "aloof" and "reserved" (Fido, 2001).

KEITH HUNTER JESPERSON

Keith Hunter Jesperson was an Oregan long haul trucker who was suspected of 136 killings. He scrolled a string of taunting confessions like this one on a road stop restroom walls "I killed Tanya Bennett . . I beat her to death, raped her, and loved it. Yes I am sick, but I enjoy myself too" (Schindehette, 2005).

JAVED IGBAL

Javed Igbal mutilated and savagely killed hundreds of street children and put them into acid (Morrison and Goldberg, 2004). He then completed suicide, which is interesting as it is often stated that "serial murderers rarely commit suicide".

Vinnie Connell

In Ireland, Michael Sheridan wrote a book called *Frozen Blood: Psycho and Serial Killers in Ireland* Gerry O'Carroll with Michael Sheridan has written an autobiography published by Penguin Books on the same topic. In *Frozen Blood,* Sheridan puts forward a controversial theory that "serial killers could be responsible for a number of women in Ireland" (Murphy, 2004).

Sheridan (2003) in discussing the late Vinnie Connell describes him as a disc jockey who was anti-woman. He strangled women. He had huge empathy deficits. He "beat up his mother" and tortured other women according to Sheridan. He had ferocious temper tantrums. He was an extremely controlling person. He had autistic charm and was for a period "a lay preacher". He was a Jekyll and Hyde figure. He had identity diffusion and multiple selves. As well as being violent, he was also an arsonist. Like a number of serial killers, he worked for a time as a "policeman" It is difficult to know how many he killed according to Sheridan, but he wrote that "Detective Gerry O'Carroll has no doubt that this evil genius could have been responsible for the death of at least half a dozen women" He had Criminal Autistic Psychopathy.

Killers of US Presidents, Political Leaders, Celebrities (Criminal Autistic Pyschopathy), and Schools

These killers often have Autistic Psychopathy as indeed do single handed killers in schools.

Julies Charles Guiteau

Julies Charles Guiteau shot the President of the United States. He had great difficulty separating fact from fiction. He possessed very poor life skills and was taken to court for debt. He killed the President because he did not make him an Ambassador to Paris. In court he conducted his own defence which is typical enough for persons with Criminal Autistic Psychopathy. This is a typical autistic defensive position. He was not a serial killer. (Nash, 197.)

John Wilkes Booth

John Wilkes Booth possibly had Criminal Autistic Psychopathy (Nash, 1975). He was a rich actor. He was obsessed with being remembered as a significant figure. He was described as an eccentric. Both of these features are associated with Criminal Autistic Psychopathy. He shot Abraham Lincoln. He was not a serial killer.

OTHER KILLERS

Robert Francois Damiens

One could ask the question, but of course there is no proof that Robert Francois Damiens, who attempted in 1757 to kill Louis XV was executed by a slow savage process, had Criminal Autistic Psychopathy. He seemed to be "immune from pain; he had his head raised and watched the proceedings with curiosity, and when the lead was poured into the wounds cried "more, more!" (Wilson, 1971). Persons with Criminal Autistic Psychopathy sometimes have very low sensitivity to pain and are fearless.

Jesse Pomeroy

Jesse Pomeroy was regarded as a serial killer long before that term became popular and indeed he antedated Jack the Ripper in England (Wilson, 1971). He mutilated and killed children. They were strangled and tortured. Like many serial killers with Criminal Autistic Psychopathy, they were buried in his home. He killed about 27 in all. He was full of anger, rage, and hatred.

Ludwig Tessnov

In the latter part of the 19th century and early 20th century, Ludwig Tessnov killed and mutilated quite a number of boys and girls. This happened in Rugen in the Baltic region. (Wilson. 1971).

Nicklaus Stuller

An example of a lust murder happened in 1577 by Nicklaus Stuller who was written up by Hans Schmidt in the Journal of Master Hans Schmidt (Keller, 1928). According to Wilson, Schmidt wrote that "first he shot a horse-soldier; secondly he cut open a pregnant woman alive in which was a dead child; thirdly he again cut open a pregnant woman in whom was a female child; fourthly he once more cut open a pregnant woman in whom were two male children" (Wilson, 1977). This has echoes of Criminal Autistic Psychopathy.

According to Wilson in a *Hang Man's Diary* edited by Albrecht Keller, 1928, there is mention of a case where according to Wilson a man "broke into a mill and shot the miller, raped the wife and the maid, then made the wife fry eggs and beat them off the body of her husband."

Andreas Bichel

Richard von Krafft-Ebing (1965) discusses the case of Andreas Bichel. "He killed and dissected the ravished girls." With reference to one of his victims, at his examination he expressed himself as follows: "I opened her breast and with a knife cut through the fleshy parts of the body. Then I arranged the body as a butcher does beef, and hacked it with an axe into pieces of a size to fit the whole which I had dug up in the mountains for burying it. I may say that while opening the body I was so greedy that I trembled, and could have cut out a piece and eaten it."

Masters (1993) points out that Andrew Bichel "born about 1770 in Bavaria, killed young girls and handled their intestines before cutting them in half."

Case M

Krafft-Ebing (1965) discusses a man he calls Case M. who cut up a girl a child of 4 years of age and was found with the forearm of the child in his pocket and "the head and entrails, in a half-charred condition, were taken from the stove" He showed no remorse. He developed "tardily and imperfectly" in childhood. He was regarded as being evil at puberty and unattractive. He engaged in sexuality with animals. He showed "morbid changes of the frontal lobes, of the first and second temporal convolutions, and of a part of the occipital convolutions" (Krafft-Ebing, 1965)

Bacher Case

Krafft-Ebing (1965) points out that a man called Bacher operated towards the end of the 19th century in France. He strangled his victims and mutilated them. As a child he was regarded as being vicious. He sexually abused a small child when he was 20. He was very paranoid and threatening. When a girl turned him down he shot himself and produced a "facial paralysis". On the 10th of September 1896 "he committed his usual atrocity on a Mrs. Mounier, just married, 19 years of age, and on the 1st of October on Rodier, a shepherdess 14 years of age. He cut out her genitals and carried them away. Towards the end of May 1897 he killed a tramp boy, 14 years old, by cutting his throat".

In his early life, he was "vicious and fond of maltreating animals". He had a poor work record. He was not regarded as normal. "He slept badly, constantly dreamed of murder" He engaged in 11 lust murders which were sadistic. He probably had Criminal Autistic Psychopathy. He showed no remorse.

Leger Case

Krafft-Ebing (1965) described Leger as "moody, silent, and shy of people" He killed a girl, mutilated her genitals, tore out her heart, "ate a bit, drank the blood, and buried the remains". He was callous and showed no guilt. He was executed. He was not a serial killer, but showed features characteristic of serial killers.

Tirsch Case

In the late 1800s, Krafft-Ebing (1965) describes Tirsch as a man who disliked women. He killed a woman, mutilated her body, and cooked her at home and in the course of the next few days ate her. He was described as a silent, peculiar, coarse, very irritable, grumbling and revengeful man. He was an outsider and wanted execution. He was not a serial killer or more likely was caught before he could progress to serial killing. He probably had Criminal Autistic Psychopathy.

Vincenz Verzeni

Krafft-Ebing (1965) also describes Vincenz Verzeni born in 1849. He strangled people and mutilated the people that he killed. He also sexually abused them. He was of average intelligence and was described as being peculiar "silent, and inclined to be solitary" and had a large head. His acts involved ejaculation. "As soon as he had grasped his victim by the neck, sexual sensations were experienced".

Verzeni sucked blood from his victims. He roasted some of their flesh at home. He stated that he was under an impulse that he could not control and had a high sex drive. He was a lust killer. He felt very relaxed and contented after a killing. He had no guilt, no remorse, and no evidence of conscience. He sucked his victim's blood. He pointed out that if he was let out of prison, he would murder more as he had irresistible impulses. Killing sexually aroused him enormously. He had a heightened sense of smell particularly the "clothing and intestines" of victims. He had Criminal Autistic Psychopathy.

Sergeant Bertrand

Krafft-Ebing (1965) also discusses Sergeant Bertrand who was a peculiar character and "from childhood silent and inclined to solitude". He seemed to have very powerful sexual impulses. He fantasised about killing and having sex with people. First, he began interacting with animals where "he would cut open the abdomen, tear out the entrails, and masturbate during the act. He declared that in this way he experienced inexpressible pleasure" He then began digging up bodies in graveyards. He would cut open the bodies and masturbate. He was a compulsive masturbator. He had sexual intercourse with corpses. He had Criminal Autistic Psychopathy.

Ardisson

Krafft-Ebing (1965) describes another man, Ardisson born in 1872. He was also involved with dead bodies of females and "practiced cunnilingus on them". "He lived isolated by himself and was very morose" He suffered no guilt and had worked as a stonemason and as a gravedigger. He had an emotionally impoverished personality. He drank his own semen. He could not relate to girls, but drank their urine after he observed them urinating. He had no shame or guilt. He had Criminal Autistic Psychopathy. He was not a serial killer.

Lucian Staniak

The Polish multiple killer Lucian Staniak killed, raped, and mutilated the bodies. He killed about 20 people (Leyton, 1989).

The Case of DW

The Necrophilia case DW "he was never married and states that he has always been very shy in the company or presence of young women. He was a confirmed masturbator". (De River, 1956). When his girlfriend died "he felt the urge to jump into the casket with her, and he actually wanted to be buried alive with his sweetheart". De River (1956) noted that "he does not make friends easily and does not care to. He is antisocial". He was a student of history and he also enjoys all works of psychological nature. He drank a corpses blood and it excited him. He "sucked the urine from the bladder of a corpse" and this excited him He interfered with hundreds of corpses. He was an embalmer. He had Criminal Autistic Psychopathy.

Alfred Fish

Alfred Fish killed and ate a child (Morrison et al, 2004). Fish was said to be an emotionless prisoner who, when interviewed by detectives explained that he had "a thirst for blood". He showed evidence of autistic novelty seeking and experimentation on the body. He was also very masochistic and inserted needles between his scrotum and rectum. Being executed in the electric chair was a novelty for him and he looked forward to this new experience.

"Alfred Fish was tried for murder, but it was his necrophilia which drew attention to him. His victims were children, and the body of one little child was used to make stew" (Masters, 1993). He had Criminal Autistic Psychopathy.

Mark James Robert Essex

Mark James Robert Essex was not a traditional serial killer. (Leyton, 1989) He had a happy childhood, but later suffered vicious and severe racism while in the Navy. This radicalised him and led him to develop a hatred of whites of whom he began to kill in one killing spree. He killed mainly white police officers. They finally caught him and cornered him. He had 200 bullet holes in his body from the police etc.. He was a man who suffered deep narcissistic wounds in the navy. He left behind him "10 dead, 22 wounded, and millions of dollars worth of property in ruins" (Leyton, 1989).

His first killing was on New Years Eve 1972 then he finally took on the whole Police Department with officers from surrounding areas as he was holed up in a Hotel setting fires and shooting at white police officers. His school record was average, but he was good at technical subjects and did well on the entrance to the Navy. He was court-martialled and fined in the Navy for a trumped up charge of playing music too loudly. The second time he could not take the racism and went abroad without leave and was court-martialled on his return and punished. He was a man with a cause. This is totally different from serial killers described in this book where the killing is often for pleasure.

THE ARTS AND CRIMINAL AUTISTIC PSYCHOPATHY

Mary Shelley's Frankenstein

In typical Criminal Autistic Psychopathy fashion, Frankenstein was born without a theory of mind, without a capacity for empathy and he had to observe the world and model himself and imitate the world. Mary Shelley says about Frankenstein that he was solitary and abhorrent. He was a very inhumane character who was unhappy with his odd face.

Robert Shroud: The Birdman of Alcatraz

While Robert Shroud was a multiple murderer but not a serial killer, he had Criminal Autistic Psychopathy.

According to Gaddis (1985) Robert Shroud was in solitary confinement for 39 years. Although he murdered two males "he was eligible for parole in 1936". Probably he did not get it because he challenged the prison system and got married while in prison. Anyone who challenges the system has to be viciously punished and this was done by the American Department of Justice and the prison system in America in relation to Robert. He showed a lack of "cop on" in challenging the system in the way he did and becoming a national figure opposed to them.

He clearly had Criminal Autistic Psychopathy and an autistic superego. It was an autistic superego and a sense of injustice which lead him to kill the first man who beat up his girlfriend and the second man who was a prison guard / thug in the prisons. It was not that he had low standards it was that his standards were too high and his sense of injustice too great. His actions were culturally inappropriate and indeed inappropriate at other levels as well.

Robert's father was an abusive angry man who abused alcohol. His father often beat him. At four years of age he was "an abstracted, lonely boy" (Gaddis, 1985). This is typical of persons with Criminal Autistic Psychopathy. He had poor peer relationships in school, was a poor mixer, was an isolated child, and suffered depression. He had very poor social skills. He was a daydreamer.

Robert was fearless. He was friendless in relation to the neighbourhood children. He spent time as an autistic wanderer. This was in later adolescence. He had awkward physical movements. He was a boy with enormous persistence and he showed this in adult life as well. He had a narrow focus. He worked initially as an electrician a kind of work attractive to those with Criminal Autistic Psychopathy.

When he shot a man he immediately went and gave himself up and confessed everything. This is also fairly typical. The man he killed had abused his girlfriend. In prison he was withdrawn "with eyes as hard as a blue china plate" (Gaddis, 1985). He began to study mathematics and was an autodictat. He had clearly mathematical talent. He identified himself as an outsider and identified himself with the prisoners. Scientific matters fascinated him but also by more strange topics like theosophy.

Persons with Autistic Psychopathy are often fascinated by these strange topics and by the occult. He also studied engineering. He was a very intelligent man. His problems were in the social emotional arena. He then killed a vicious prison guard. This led to him going into solitary and being sentenced to death, which was commuted by the President after the intercession of his mother with the President Wilson's wife. The prison guard was abusive and again Shroud's autistic superego overwhelmed him. Psychiatrists found Robert very odd and eccentric and unclassifiable at the time.

Persons with Autistic Psychopathy often have odd beliefs and Shroud had the belief that "he could send mental messages beyond the walls" (Gaddis, 1985). These kinds of ideas are not uncommon in Autistic Psychopathy (Abell and Hare, 2005). He was a great observer as persons with Autistic Psychopathy often are. He studied music and began composing. He had an enormous memory. He found solitary confinement in a way relatively easy for him because it allowed him to focus on his narrow interests. Of course it became tedious as the years went by. He did some painting there as well. Then he found some sparrows in the exercise yard and began to care for them and developed this massive interest in birds and particularly canaries and became one of the greatest experts on canaries and canaries' illnesses in America and identified some new veterinary conditions that affected them.

People wrote to him from all over America asking for advice on sick canaries. He wrote a book on this that was published. His mother began to sell the canaries that he was rearing and he contributed to magazines on canaries.

Robert had what Gaddis describes as "an accurate memory, amounting to almost total visual recall; and limitless patience" (Gaddis, 1985). He was meticulous about keeping his hands clean. His bird keeping had a good effect on the rest of the prison and seemed to calm it down and other prisoners began to take an interest in various kinds of things, which helped as well. He was hungry for knowledge and was always learning as autodictats always are. He discovered a cure for "septic fever in birds" (Gaddis, 1985).

His great support (his mother) was upset when he married a woman, Della Jones, with an interest in birds. His mother then withdrew from him and indeed was heartbroken and died shortly afterwards. In a way it was tactless to do this, as his mother hated this new woman. He also grossly alienated the Department of Justice and the prison authorities with this marriage.

Over the various times of his imprisonment, he became a "cause celeb" and there were huge efforts to get him released. J. Edgar Hoover Head of the FBI visited him. Later he studied law in prison. He was in a number of prisons, but Alcatraz was the most famous on an island off San Francisco. He died in prison.

HAROLD SHIPMAN

Harold Shipman was the most prolific ever-serial killer in UK history. Damien Thompson (2005) in a review of C. Peter's book *Harold Shipman* wrote in an article titled *"How the addicted angel of death winged it for so long"* in *Ireland on Sunday*, Thompson points out that he killed over 250 patients making him the second most prolific serial killer in the history after Pedro Lopez the so-called "monster of the Andes" Thompson (2005) points out that "in one little cul-de-sac, he killed six elderly ladies" (and) "it was not unknown for two pensioners to die on one day". Thompson quotes Carol Peter's (2005) comment that he was "a psychopath who enjoyed playing god" He was a very devious person and talked prison officers into a false sense of security before he completed suicide. The final triggering factor for suicide was a reduction of privileges in prison, which he found narcissistically wounding.

Background

Shipman was not a great student at school and had to re-sit many exams. He showed very odd behaviour at Medical School where he showed a typical fascination with dead bodies. He was "fascinated with corpses" liked touching them and "stayed in the hospital morgue after the other students had gone home". The fascination and the thrill of the dead body was already there. Peters (2005) noted that an old acquaintances always experienced "this emotional distancing" by him and when he came to attention with his behaviour he wanted nothing to do with people from his early life".

Studholme (2005) notes that "he was always on the fringe, but he placed himself on the fringe". This is typical of Autistic Psychopathy. He was an "outsider" during school days. Bob goes on to state that "he was a man of few words . . very determined . . he had a real streak of ruthlessness" . His mother died of cancer shortly after receiving a morphine injection from her GP. This did not make him a serial killer as people have believed. This is simplistic socio-babble so popular with the "chattering classes" Harold Shipman replied to a question from a classmate Michael Health which was autistic in its form and brevity. Heath asked "was there anything exciting at the weekend Fred?". Fred replied "no" "my mum died" When she died, he went out onto the street and ran for hours "in the middle of the night". Here instead of thinking about the psychic pain of grief, he went and acted it out by running. It showed a very poor capacity for emotional processing. It was a grossly abnormal acute grief reaction. This was genetically underpinned behaviour - not learned behaviour. Killing was later part of that acting out behaviour, as was being a drug addict.

Social Relationships

For Shipman there was only one person in the world and that was himself. Everybody else were just objects to be used. (Rogers *et al*, 2004). In prison, he showed "no regard for anyone apart from himself" He was contemptuous and superior to everybody else in prison, and of course that related in the same way to victims' families. He dismissed the excellent person who led his public enquiry as "Dame Edna" He was full of bile and hatred. He was very narcissistic and grandiose. He showed gross empathy deficits and deficits in reciprocal social relations according to Rogers *et al* (2004). His letters show "a supremely conceited and sinister man, who sees those around him as "low grade ore" or "very poor quality manure". He dehumanised people and saw himself as superman and people in general as "almost vermin".

The victims had no right to challenge the great man. This has a very strong Nazi flavour, reminiscent of the Nazi extermination activities before and during the 2nd World War. He showed "a callous indifference to death" of victims. His only interest was in the excitement of killing. Britton (1995) also suggested that Harold's "sexual fulfilment is intensely cerebral and mental experience with no physical contact necessary". Peters (2005) notes that as a child "he did not play out" His characteristics are all classic symtoms of a person with Criminal Autistic Psychopathy. He was an unempathic serial killer.

Language and Non-verbal Behaviour

Britton (1995) noted that "he talked to himself in the third person". He also showed an arrogant tone of voice. He wrote 10,000 letters to a friend - Shirley Horsfall. Persons with Autistic Psychopathy (a subgroup of Asperger's syndrome) are great letter writers. The letters often show Semantic Pragmatic difficulties in expression or an autistic narrative and are very difficult to follow (Rogers *et al*, 2004).

Control

Peters (2005) quotes Brian Whittle as stating "Fred (Shipman) himself was a terrific disciplinarian."

Rogers *et al* (2004) note that he wrote from prison "as I am not in charge there is very little I can do (to) affect anyone's actions" This is central to his upset with the prison system. He was a man who always wanted to dominate, to control, and to tell people what to do.

Identity Diffusion

Identity diffusion is critical to Criminal Autistic Psychopathy. Shipman had an uncertain identity all his life, being seen as the good doctor and the loss of this devastated him. He suffered from identity diffusion. He had no authentic core.

Criminal Autistic Psychopathic Novelty Seeking

Britton told Peters (2005) that "the thrills that are associated with killing and the sense of peacefulness at the end would have been more intense in his younger days". Shipman had therefore to increase the killings to get the same buzz. We can only speculate that he had the so-called "novelty seeking gene" in great abundance e.g. Dopamine D4 polymorphism. His drug addiction to pethedine from medical school was possibly part of the same process. His drug abuse as a Doctor came to the attention of the controlling authorities.

Profile

Prison letters revealed Shipman's last crises. *Sunday Times,* January 18, 2005, they say he was "a calculating and sadistic character". He developed an alternative façade to cover for his killing. He was community worker and visited his patients at home. He was tremendously energetic as people with Autistic Psychopathy often are. He appears to have no conscience and no remorse and had no capacity to see other people as human beings. To keep getting his high, he had to kill more frequently as he got older. He had to increase the danger level to get his high, for example, altering a patient's will before killing. In hospital training, he had poor social relationships particularly with authority. He tended to humiliate people. Harold decided who was to live and who was to die. He was like God! In prison he probably suffered from depression. According to Roger and Ungoed-Thomas (2004), Shipman was given what he called "happy pills" - most likely anti-depressants.

The Criminal Medical Autistic Psychopathy

Shipman picked "soft targets" for his killings. He was a coward. He was caught when he falsified a will of a patient that he killed. He made himself the sole beneficiary. He felt himself omnipotent, god like. It was also partly to increase the thrill and the perversity of the killing, in that not alone did he rob the woman of her life, he also robbed her of her money. Britton (1995) describes Shipman as being "aloof, cold, calculating, self-centred, grandiose . . arrogant" Shipman was the Hyde of Jekyll and Hyde or indeed he was both Jekyll and Hyde the good doctor and the vicious killer. Rogers *et al* (2004) describe him as a "cold blooded killer".

Murphy(2004) pointed out that "on the other side of the caring husband, community activist, or quite intelligent neighbour is a cold, sadistic grandiose" killer.

Sokol (2004) states "that Fred was a very popular among his patients. They loved his endearing bedside manner and his willingness to visit patients at home. Some called him the best doctor in the region" He showed typical Autistic Psychopathic charisma. He was a great liar. He was addicted to killing. The power of death gave him great thrills and to maintain the thrill he had to kill more frequently as he got older.

When he completed suicide, people stated that "he had removed our hopes of finding out why he did it". (Herbert *et al,* 2004). The reason he killed was for pleasure because he had Criminal Autistic Psychopathy.

TED BUNDY

"For murder, though it have no tongue, will speak with most miraculous organ". (Hamlet)

Ted Bundy said, "I'm a psychologist, and it really gives me insight". (in Leyton, 1989).

Ted Bundy was a psychologist, counsellor, and a devious serial killer who disposed of probably more than 36 women. He showed no empathy or guilt. He killed his victims with an iron bar. On occasion he had one future victim watch another victim being killed. (Depue and Schindehette, 2005).

Bundy, when on death row in the state prison in Stark Florida, "was the most calculating and cunning of all the serial killers". "Bundy talked about how in one dual murder, he kept one victim alive so she could see her friend being killed. He talked about clubbing his victims with a crowbar, handcuffing them, and then chatting with them when they regained consciousness just for sport. The one thing he never expressed was remorse" (Depue and Schindehette, 2005).

It is not true that persons with Criminal Autistic Psychopathy cannot be as calculating as some naïve professionals believe.

Bundy is a classic example of the organised personality. Sometimes killers go back to the scene of the crime. For some, "it is the urge to relive the pleasure of the crime, which is so powerful it outweighs even the fear of being apprehended".

Personal History

At college he got a Bachelors Degree in Psychology and then went on the study Law but did not complete the course. He worked for a period as a Crisis Counsellor. A colleague of his at the Crisis Counselling Centre, according to Leyton, stated that he "always seemed to respond to the callers with sort of a cold lecture, telling them they should learn to discipline their emotions, to take charge. He did not seem to have . . the compassion, the understanding that these people were unable to take control" (Depue and Schindehette, 2005). This is the type of counselling persons with Autistic Psychopathy give. This was because of his lack of empathy. He was regarded as being a very strange person.

In College he related poorly to people. He became interested in the law as persons with Autistic Psychopathy often are because of its rather cut and dried nature, and its dependence on precedence and what's written down. A lot of it is text based which persons with Autistic Psychopathy like.

He was a republican political party supporter and activist. He spent a period at law school. He was fascinated by police and law work as many serial killers are. He was interested in police activities and indeed pretended to be a policeman on one occasion. He was highly intelligent. He was described as being extremely shy. This was in childhood. He had identity diffusion.

He wanted to control and dominate people. He had problems in intimacy with females. He was a novelty seeker and a risk taker. He was narcissistic, grandiose, and exhibitionistic. He lacked guilt.

He used to steal from shops earlier in life. He had one period where he was engaged to be married, but could not go through with it any further and went off. It was at this time and before the engagement was terminated that he began to murder. (Leyton, 1989).

Features of Autistic Psychopathy

Bundy had an autistic charisma. He was perverse, egocentric, narcissistic, voyeuristic, exhibitionistic and sadistic. He had very poor intimate relationships. He totally lacked empathy. He had no sense how his victims felt. It is not certain how many people he murdered. Some estimates put it almost at 100 according to Ann Rule. He was obsessed by domination and control, and showed an autistic need to control. He constantly changed his legal advisors or often sacking them something that probably hastened his journey to the electric chair. This is typical of persons with Criminal Autistic Psychopathy.

We have little information about his biological father even though this is critical information. He was extremely shy. He was teased and bullied. He was egocentric and introverted. He was into minor criminal activities early in life. He was somewhat of a linguist. He spoke about the killer within him the killer self in the third person, which is not uncommon in persons with Criminal Autistic Psychopathy. He also tended to make brief autistic communications and speak in the autistic narrative style.

Bundy engaged in a kind of autistic narrative with the police, which was difficult to follow. His sentences were vague not having clear context and difficult to understand. He blamed others for his problems and for his incarceration. He blamed the State. He played with words in Court and was fascinated by words and trying to outwit the prosecution. He had poor social interactional skills early in life but did develop a kind of pseudonormality or false self later in life. Persons with Criminal Autistic Psychopathy can be fascinated by language and can learn how to show a false or pseudo self.

He was always naïve. He was always immature. In a way he was also a loner type personality. The world had to adapt to him and he was never willing to adapt to the world.

He could show a pseudowarmth and he was a cold personality. He was contemptuous of all authority that is psychologists, psychiatrists, police officers, and the judiciary as well as juries. He felt himself to be superior to them and blamed them constantly for making mistakes. He could play the pseudo normal role and therefore people were surprised that he had this other life. People found it impossible to really know him. This is typical of Criminal Autistic Psychopathy.

Ted Bundy was regarded as a good psychology college student. Because of his high IQ he was able to develop social strategies to deal with his intimacy and close personal relationships difficulties. He abused alcohol. His non-verbal behaviour was noted to be "wooden and rigid" (Leyton, 1989).

He was also a rather snobbish individual. He feared real intimacy with a live woman. He was aware of his deficits in social interpersonal skills. Like many narcissistic grandiose people he was contemptuous of the police initially. The same would go for Harold Shipman. He was antiauthority and hostile to authority and to newspapermen. He was a chameleon like figure in terms of identity. He had some insight in that what he was doing probably had genetic underpinnings. He found it hard to deal with unstructured social situations in College.

According to Simon (1996), Ted Bundy "choose young women who parted their long hair down the middle of their head" He liked to prolong the killings and would allow victims to regain consciousness for further discussions before finally dispatching them. Prolonging the killing episode increased his sadistic thrill. Bundy said as he killed he was aware that "you feel the last bit of breath leaving their body. You look into their eyes. A person in that situation is god! (Simon, 1996). He went on to state "you then possess them and they shall be part of you, and the grounds where you kill them or leave them becomes sacred to you, and you will always be drawn back to them".

Ted Bundy killed because he wanted to kill. He had Criminal Autistic Psychopathy with a high IQ. He was well capable of lying although many professionals believe that persons with this condition cannot lie. Bundy was an organised killer, except towards the end of his killing when he became careless and disorganised. Simon (1996) points out that a serial killer was callous, schizoid, and unsociable.

Ted Bundy is probably the most infamous psychologist ever. Ann Rule did counselling with him at a Centre in the United States. He was a Jekyll and Hyde character. He had many separate compartments in his mind that did not communicate. He was addicted to murder. He strangled as his instrument to kill and sexually abused victims. He was extremely self-destructive. He was attractive to women and many women were attracted to him. Clearly he was completely disloyal to them and would have relationships with a number of women at the same time. He married after being imprisoned and somehow managed to have a daughter. He was extremely devious and a tremendous liar. His behaviour could not be explained on environmental grounds or due to childhood traumas although there were some. He tended to steal things. He was indecisive. He used and abused people. He did suffer personal rejections probably before he started his killing. These were simply precipitants to the killing. He was particularly interested in murdering university type women who parted their hair in the middle. Once he got into killing the instinct to kill and the excitement of killing became overwhelming. He was very narcissistic and grandiose. He had deficiencies in reality testing. (Stone, 1993).

Bundy was voyeuristic. He liked the chase that is finding a woman to kill. A woman was an object, a dehumanised human being, to be used as he saw fit and for him to possess totally in death. The killing was also a self-esteem regulator an activity that improved sense of self, power, control, and gave a sense of fulfilment.

He could find nothing to do in life anything remotely as exciting as killing. He picked on vulnerable people. When he was on death row he was incredibly attractive to many women who wrote to him etc.. His lack of empathy and extreme control was shown in the court case when he would defend himself and harangued people and alienated judges and juries.

Ted Bundy saw himself as being treated by the American state in the same way that the Russian state treated their dissidents. He was very taken with the Gulag Archipelago. He saw himself as a victim like Alexander Solzhenitsyn in the Soviet Union.

There were no limits. He was a Jekyll and Hyde figure. Bundy said when sentenced to execution "I cannot accept the sentence . . . because it is not a sentence to me . . it is a sentence to someone else who is not standing here today" (Masters, 1993). This shows his identity diffusion. He had separated off here the killing self from other selves. (Masters, 1993). He was finally hanged after innumerable appeals.

A prison Psychiatrist Dr. Van O. Austin stated that Bundy "does have some features of the antisocial personality, such as a lack of guilt feelings, callousness, and very pronounced tendency to compartmentalise and methodologically rationalise his behaviour . . at times he has lived a lonely, somewhat withdrawn reclusive existence, which is consistent with . . a Schizoid Personality" (Leyton, 1989). I would call it preferably Criminal Autistic Psychopathy.

Ted Bundy said:

> "I don't feel guilty for anything . . . I feel sorry for people who feel guilt" quoted in Leyton (1989).
> "I've always felt somehow lost in my life" quoted in Leyton (1989).

TIMOTHY MCVEIGH

Timothy McVeigh bombed a government building in Oklahoma and killed one hundred and sixty eight people. As already described, this is different fromkilling.

Background

According to Michel and Herbeck, 2002, as a child Timothy was rather Hyperkinetic. He loved catalogues as persons with Autistic Psychopathy often do. He was an imaginative child. He was accident-prone as children with Autistic Psychopathy and Hyperkinetic Syndrome and had a high pain threshold. He adored "drinking pickle juice" and was also an animal lover.

He was bullied as a child and was not athletic. Timothy was fascinated by how things worked. He was mechanically minded. He was obsessed as a child with guns. He was a loner. He had identity diffusion and a sense of having multiple selves. He had a disturbance of a sense of self. According to Michel and Herbeck, (2002), his favourite television show was "Star Trek". They also point out that "McVeigh saw something of himself in each of the shows characters" and was a committed Trekkie. Persons with Autistic Psychopathy are very interested in that particular programme Star Trek. He was interested in "Data – android, show no emotion. Logic rules".

He spent periods as an autistic drifter. He was vengeful. "McVeigh saw himself as a counterpart to Luke Skywalker, the heroic Jedi knight whose successful attack on the deck star closes the film" In a way he had an almost autistic sense of justice, a primitive sense of justice. In his mind, his murderous behaviour was right and challenging the injustices of the government. He possessed narrow interests and narrow ideas.

Michel and Herbeck pointed out that McVeigh "stopped shooting frogs with his BB gun because it pained him to see the creatures suffer. Later, when he killed men in battle, he found it difficult to suppress his sense of the injustices of war". He was a great reader. "He was dark and brooding". They also described him as "cold and calculating". He was very narcissistic and egocentric. He was very controlling with poor relationship skills. For him people existed to be used by him as he pleased. He always blamed others for whatever happened. He showed lack of guilt, remorse and was extremely vengeful.

When in prison McVeigh wanted his sperm taken "out of prison" and given to a woman "so she could become pregnant". This gives some idea of his concept of a relationship

Michel and Herbeck (2002) claim that McVeigh once claimed that the government "had injected a computer chip into his buttock before the army shipped him over to Desert Storm". This sounds like a kind of autistic delusion or the kind of delusional thinking that persons with autism do have.

His father was described as the "salt of the earth". He was mathematically minded.

Timothy wore a tee-shirt saying "Thus ever to tyrants". John Wilksbooth said this when he killed Abraham Lincoln. On the back of his shirt he had a Thomas Jefferson quotation "the tree of liberty must be refreshed from time to time with the blood of patriots and tyrants". Jefferson and John WilkesBooth both had Autistic Psychopathy. McVeigh's bombing action was in retaliation for "US military actions against smaller nations".

He had Criminal Autistic Psychopathy.

WAGNER VON DEGERLOCK

Wagner von Degerlock is what one would call a spree killer and not a serial killer. In one shooting, he killed eight males, one female, and injured a dozen others. He was a 39-year-old schoolteacher. He had Criminal Autistic Psychopathy. He also murdered his family, i.e. his wife and four children. He felt persecuted and ridiculed by the inhabitants of the town of Muehlhausen where this killing spree took place. This kind of paranoid thinking is common in Criminal Autistic Psychopathy. He wanted to die and was extremely angry that he was not given the death penalty. He was a rather shy individual who according to Bruch (1967) "insisted on using High German even in his private life".

Wagner had an autistic superego and was very guilty about masturbation. He had poor reality testing. He felt that people knew and were talking about a sexual act that he engaged in at one time. There was significant marital disharmony in his marriage yet he did like his children. His own thinking was created in an autistic world, which was not tested by external reality that is killing his family to save them from a hurtful world and then taking vengeance on people who were not talking about him or making comments about him. This is typical of these autistic type delusions. He could easily have been misdiagnosed as suffering from dementia praecox or what is now called schizophrenia.

He was a great reader and also wrote poetry like many persons with Autistic Psychopathy. He was also interested in drama. He "compared himself to Shakespeare, Shiller and Goethe". This was very grandiose. Wagner was very interested in the Nazi party and later joined the party. In literature, his case is used to "illustrate that paranoia needs to be considered separate from dementia praecox, that it is not the product of some pathological process but the outcome of complex psychological reactions" I would argue that the proper diagnosis was neither of these, but was Criminal Autistic Psychopathy.

Chapter 14

CASE HISTORIES OF FEMALE KILLERS

ELIZABETH BALTHORY: HUNGARIAN COUNTESS AND FEMALE DRACULA

According to Masters and Lea (in Jones Robinson, 2002), Elizabeth Countess Balthory: Countess Dracula bathed in the blood of over 600 females, girls, and young women. She was into witchcraft and the black arts. She gathered people of this kind of persuasion around her. Children were snatched from the countryside to be killed often sadistically for the purpose of her bathing in their blood. After she bathed she got children to lick the blood off her body. Most of the victims were brought to the Countess's bed and there "bitten to death") Many of the girls were sadistically tortured before being killed. This has deep echoes of sadistic serial killing. She felt that their blood would keep her beautiful. She felt the blood would stop her growing old and remain beautiful. (Glynn Jones, 2002).

According to McNally (1983), it was reported at her trial that:

"She sometimes poured cold water over the girls, until the water turned to ice in the cold. The girls froze and died."

This is sadistic killing. At other times if she was displeased with a servant she would thrust a hot iron into the servants face until the servants "mouth, nose, and throat would become a great burning wound" (McNally, 1983). She set one servant on fire and on another occasion she "put her fingers into a sewing girl's mouth and pulled it until the girl's mouth spent at the corners" (McNally, 1983). Some of her tortures was quite prolonged and drawn out in the classic serial killing tradition. The countess was "addicted to biting human flesh" (McNally, 1983).

Like some other serial killers for example Gilles de Rais she "observed religious rituals" (McNally, 1983). Eventually she was tried and charged after she killed more aristocratic girls. She escaped the usual sentence of decapitation but was instead put under capture "castle arrest".

Bram Stoker's novel *Dracula* also had the biting and drawings of blood of humans as an important feature.

McNally notes the following words over a School of Criminal Anthropology in France "Every society has the criminals it deserves". This is a sociological view with very little relevance to serial killers who are driven by internal often innate factors.

ELIZABETH BROWNRIGG

Elizabeth Brownrigg was a murderer and midwife. She engaged in savage barbarity with pregnant women in her care. She would flog them until she had to stop through exhaustion (Glyn Jones, 2002). Another female Mary Clifford was given even more savage treatment and indeed died from the torture. On another occasion she cut a girls tongue with a scissors. Mary Clifford and another girl were frequently so beaten that their heads and shoulders appeared as one general sore; and, when a plaster was applied to their wounds, the skin use to peel away with it. At night she would keep a girl in a "coal-hole", with "hands tied behind her" and a chain "about her neck" (Glynn Jones, 2002).

She would also grab a girl by the cheeks and "forcing the skin down violently with her fingers, cause the blood to gush from her eyes" (Glynn Jones, 2002). She would torture one girl in front of another. Mrs. Brownrigg was finally caught, tried and hanged.

That she could do what she did "can only be accounted for by the depravity of human nature, which philosophers have always disputed, but which true Christians will be ready to allow" Glynn Jones, (2002).

IRMA GRESE

Irma Grese, a female Nazi "was the epitome of inhumane sadism, torture beyond belief, and extravagant murder". (Nash, in Glyn Jones, 2002). Irma Grese was "resolute, unyielding, and devoid of compassion in her SS uniform. She had innumerable ways of torturing and killing the inmates. She knew when they would be gassed and taunted them about the way they would be killed. She adored and found killing massively enjoyable. She killed prisoners with starving Alsatian dogs for her amusement. She killed women and children as a form of personal amusement. She "whipped prisoners to near death". She would shoot prisoners on whim. She arranged for "the skins of murdered prisoners made into lampshades" She had these lampshades in her house. She suffered no guilt. She regarded the people she murdered as "dreck". She would also cut women's breasts "with her whip" She was a sadistic serial killer. It is not true that only males can be sadistic serial killers (Nash, 2002).

She showed no evidence of guilt, of a conscience and showed no evidence of remorse. She was tried and hanged by the British. Evil is not an exclusively male phenomenon and neither is serial killing.

ILSE KOCH

According to Nash (in Glyn Jones, 2002), Heinrich Himmler selected Ilse Koch in a bookshop as a suitable bride for his assistant Karl Koch. After marriage she became very promiscuous. Nash states that "her appetite for sex was insatiable, and her desire for perversion and sadistic acts obsessive" She arranged for prisoners to be savagely beaten to death in front of her. She got guards to do "mass slayings" of prisoners for her amusement. She murdered prisoners as well. She had prisoners murdered for their tattooed skin, which she made into lampshades. Like Jeffrey Dahlmer she had prisoners skulls in her drawing room. She was caught and sentenced to life imprisonment, which made her only laugh.

MRS. VERMILYA: THE THRILL OF THE KILL

Smith (in Glyn Jones, 2002) describes Mrs. Vermilya as a "necrophile" If this is so, this would bring her very much into the "male serial killer arena". He states that

> "Instead of being repelled and horrified by death and the dead, she was attracted to them"
> Mrs. Vermilya's mind turned about death and the dead. Her topics of conversation revolved about the matter of who would die next. She almost kept a record of the sick in her neighbourhood, and had an uncanny way of knowing where death had struck or was about to strike. She loved to spend her time in the undertakers rooms, often doing his most disagreeable work gratis." Smith (2002)

She killed many people. Death followed her everywhere or more accurately she instituted death. She killed children as well as adults. She was fascinated with death and with dead bodies. She showed no evidence of conscience, guilt or remorse. She used arsenic. After death:

> "She would appear at the end of people's rooms and seems to delight in performing those dread auspices which men must harden themselves to endure. She came and took part in the processes of preparing bodies for burial, though she usually received no pay for her work, and though she was sometimes made to feel unwelcome."

She is close enough to the sadistic male serial killer type.

JEANNE WEBBER

Lindsay (in Glyn Jones, 2002) pointed out that Jeanne Webber is a true serial killer. She chocked the children. She craved killing.

> "She killed for the pleasure of killing, and that is as unusual in murderesses as it is in murderers."

This would make her a serial killer. She was addicted to killing in France. She suffered no guilt, no remorse, and showed no evidence of conscience.

Vera Renczi: A Basement of Murdered Men

Jones (2002) was of the opinion that **Vera Renczi** was a very rebellious woman who tolerated no opposition. She always got what she wanted. She was very egocentric and narcissistic. Her husband rejecting her triggered her killing behaviour. She killed him and put him in a zinc coffin in the basement.

She began to kill men and husbands and put them in the basement. Eventually she had 35 down there. When a man wanted to leave her this upset her greatly so she "dropped a fatal dose of arsenic, adding a grain or two of strychnine for good measure. Then she callously watched him die in agony" (O'Donnell (2002). There is an element here of sadistic serial killing and not being able to deal with separations with a lover. Indeed she put it very well:

> "I could not bear to think that they might love another woman…I dare not let them go to the embraces of anyone else…". (O'Donnell in Glyn Jones, 2002).

Some male serial killers have had this same issue with separation. She would go down to her cellar where all the bodies were and she said:

> "I liked to go down there in the evenings and sit among my victims gloating over their fate" (O'Donnell (2002).

There is a necrophiliac element here. She also put her son there. She had a very high sex drive, was a fantasist, without guilt, remorse or conscience. O'Donnell noted that:

> "giving a man and a woman equally devoid of moral character, I believe the woman will usually be found to be more cruel."

It is often stated that when confronted with a group of male and female terrorists that in battle the women should be shot first because they are more fanatical and more determined. Nevertheless, males commit the great majority of crimes.

Mary Ann Cotton

Mary Ann Cotton was "Britain's mass murderess" She killed many husbands with arsenic as well as children. (O'Donnell, in Glyn Jones, 2002). She killed about 20. Some of these killings were for the purpose of financial gain, which would put these killings into acquisitive killings for gain. She killed eight of her own children and seven stepchildren. This suggests a perverse element to it and that she was addicted to killing. When she was caught she was hanged.

Helene Jegado

Emsley (2002) describes Helene Jegado (1803 – 1854) as very much a serial killer, and she killed about 30 people. It appears that she killed purely for the pleasure of killing and watching people having slow deaths. This makes her a female serial killer. She worked in various houses and when she arrived people began to die as she poisoned them with arsenic. She was finally discovered and executed.

BELLE GUINNESS

Kelleher and Kelleher (1998) stated that Belle Guinness was a Norwegian black widow who murdered something between 16 and 50 people including husbands, children, and workers. She was originally from Norway but did this murdering in America. Like many male murderers she buried the victims in her house. She was called the want add killer. She linked up with men through want ads and then killed them for their money. She "chopped up" their bodies. She burned a woman and her children as well. She killed by poisoning. She was a multiple killer who mostly killed for profit. She was not a serial killer as defined in this book.

MARIE BESNARD

Another poisoner and multiple murderer was the black widow Marie Besnard who was French and specialised in poisoning her victims for financial gain. She was never convicted and appeared to have committed the so-called "perfect crime" She murdered about 13 people (Kelleher and Kelleher, 1998).

THE GIGGLING GRANDMA

The giggling grandma was another poisoner who disposed of four husbands for financial gain. She was active from the age of about 20 to just under 50 years (Kelleher and Kelleher, 1998). She murdered 10 people including some of her own children and her mother. She was a multiple killer but not a serial killer as defined in this book. Kelleher and Kelleher (1998) point out that she was named the "giggling grandma" because of her nervous habit of giggling when discussing her crimes. She received a life imprisonment sentence. Murder for profit is a more common feature of the female multiple killer. It is uncommon for a female killer to cut up a person and eat them even though it has happened.

OTHER FEMALE MULTIPLE MURDERERS

Other female multiple murderers for profit according to Kelleher and Kelleher (1998) include Ann Marie Hahan, a German immigrant to the United States who poisoned her victims for financial gain and was executed. Antoinette Scieri murdered well over 12 for financial gain. Poison again was her method. She was originally of Italian descent. The Russian madam Popova murdered by poison about 300 males and would dispose of husbands at the request of unhappy wives. Lila Gladys Young according to Kelleher *et al* murdered over 100 infants. She would invite unmarried mothers to her home she had set up and then for a fee promised to have the babies adopted. They were more often than not killed. A female killing team Amelia Sach and Annie Walters killed infants by poisoning basically for profit. They took infants and agreed to have them adopted for a fee but killed them.

Chapter 15

CONCLUSION

It is likely that serial killing has been with us since time immemorial. While it is well identified in the United States, England, Russia, Brazil, Germany and France, it is less well identified and formally described in some other countries. It appears that it is a universal phenomenon. It is a universal psychopathological state, though very rare, it is very real. This book provides a profile of this psychopathological state.

It is inevitable that such a complex organ as the brain and the human genome will malfunction to produce serial killers only rarely. It is not unlikely that there may be some negative environmental inputs as well – certainly they are significant environmental, particularly family stresses in the histories of serial killers.

While there is a general serious and legitimate pessimism about the rehabilitation of established serial killers, there is hope that we might be able to identify children at an early stage who may have this potential. In clinical practice one often hears a mental health professional state "I am afraid he will become a killer" Indeed mothers have made the same statement often to me. The children and adolescents they are speaking about are children with severe conduct problems, empathy deficits, aggressivity, who have been suspended from school and have failed standard psychosocial treatment interventions.

I believe the psychosocial interventions should be changed in the future to efforts to help these children develop mind reading skills, empathy training, especially training in the capacity to read non-verbal behaviour. It is probable that it is easier to improve the capacity to read non-verbal behaviour at an earlier rather than a later age. The children need the strategies developed for children with Autistic Psychopathy to help them.

Up to now the psychopathology of the serial killer was inadequately characterised. This has made it very difficult to plan treatment strategies. Psychopharmacology is also going to have a critical role. Many of the serial killers will have had a past and possibly present history of Attention Deficit Hyperactivity Disorder which will need treatment with Methylphenidate or Atomoxetine. In addition they will need their severe Conduct Disorder or dangerous impulsivity treated with medications like Risperidone. Their overactive psychic system which require killing as a stimulation needs to be damped down and a combination of stimulant or Atomoxetine plus a drug like Risperidone might do this. Whether there are grounds for a depot neuroleptics is unclear.

I hope that new drugs will be developed to suppress the perverse sadistic novelty seeking or sensation seeking traits of serial killers. There are certainly cases on record where serial killers were discharged without any treatment or indeed with it and then they immediately went back to killing. We have to think in terms of prevention as there is usually a long history of fantasy, and other crimes before the period of serial killing gets into full swing which is more common in the mid 20s to the mid 30s. This may account for some early identification.

In medicine we tend to start with the most serious situations with an actual serial killer and then as time goes on we recognise more minor cases or persons who have stopped short of killing or in the fantasy stage of development. While we have many histories looking backwards there are no substitutes for prospective studies. We need to know how many adolescents with these adolescent sadistic fantasies go on to kill and are there extra factors in this switch over from the fantasy of killing to actual killing? The situation may look very different when we look at the situation prospectively rather than retrospectively as we are doing now and have no other choice because of lack of data.

It is important that we do not fall into the errors that Sigmund Freud and the Psychoanalysts made by developing analytic theories about adult psychopathology using retrospective childhood histories. The best understanding we can come up with at the moment is that serial killing is an empathy disorder, with some on the autistic spectrum. If this hypothesis is correct we would expect neurobiological deficits similar to Autistic Psychopathy as well as genetic, neuroimaging, neurochemical, hormonal, and neuropsychological deficits to be found.

The kind of potential children that I have seen clinically and considered are rare, no more than 1 in 300 of the patients referred to a Child Psychiatric Centre. These kind of numbers would be manageable from a research point of view but require very large base populations to recruit from. Up to now there has been a tendency for hopelessness and helplessness in discussions of serial killers in relation to treatment. It is helpful to distinguish the serial killers from Hitler's willing executioners, low level Civil Servants, who participated in the Holocaust by shooting Jewish adults and children. The vast majority of these did not have Criminal Autistic Psychopathy.

ADDITIONAL TABLES

Table 4.

Neurochemistry and hormones	Criminal Psychopathy	General Psychopathy
Serotonin.	50 % increased Serotonin in autism (? No increase in Criminal Autistic Psychopathy)	Reduced serontoninergic function.
MAO (Monamine oxidase).	Normal.	Low.
Noradrenaline.	Studies show low and high. ? Criminal Autistic Psychopathy.	Low.
Cortisol.	Reduced or normal.	Low.
Testosterone.	Normal.	High.
Lutenizing.	Blunted response to L.H. Stimulation in autism.	High levels of L.H. in persons demonstrating signifcant sexual aggression.

Table 5. Male/Female Brains (Norms)

	Male	Female
Amygdala.	Larger in men.	
Hippocampus.		Larger in females.
Disgust and reaction to rotting animal.	Great activity right hemisphere amygdala.	Great activity left amygdala.
Long range connectivity of the brain.		Greater in females.
Corpus callosum.		Larger in females.
Hippocampal cells.		Female hippocampal cells less damaged by chronic stress.
Verbal tasks		Better in females.
Dexterity tasks.	Better in males.	
Spatial task map reading.	Better in males.	
White matter of brain.	Males more than females.	
Number of neurons in brain.	Males have more and they are more densely packed.	
Short range connectivity in brain.	Greater in males.	
Empathy.		Females better.
Systematising.	Males better.	

Table 6.

Gender and Violence/Murder/Serial Killers	Criminal Autistic Psychopathy	General Psychopathy
Murder.	More male.	More male.
Serial killers.	More male.	More male.
Empathy.	Low males and females.	Low males and females.
Methods of killing.	? Females more poisoners Males-kill by strangulation, stabbing etc.	Females tend to be poisoners. Males kill by strangulation, stabbing etc.
Motivation.	Males kill for pleasure. Females kill mostly for financial gain but sometimes for pleasure.	Males kill in argument or for gain.. Females kill mostly for financial gain but sometimes for pleasure.
Identity.	Identity diffusion in males and females.	Identity diffusion in males and females.
Relationship to victim.	Tend to be unknown to serial killer in males. Female killers tend to know their victims.	Tend to be known to serial killer in males. Female killers tend to know their victims.
Social relationships.	Tend to be loners male and female.	Tend to be loners male and female.
Organised/disorganised killers.	Male and female organised serial killers.	Male and female organised killers.

Table 7.

	Interests	Childhood	Relationships	Behaviour
R Shroud	Mathematics, canaries	In school 'abstracted lonely boy,' autodictat.	Poor mixer, loner.	Murderer.
Marquis de Sade	Perversions, writing, novelists, playwright, science, mathematics	Poor school performance.	He abused people and lacked empathy.	Sexual abuse.
G Young	Model aeroplanes, occult, the Nazis, poisoning.	Not interested in the school curriculum, 'the mad professor'	Shy, socially awkward.	Poisoner.
T Bundy	Psychology, law, police work.	Good student.	Autistic charisma, lack of empathy and poor social relationships.	Sadistic serial killer.
P Kurten	Cruelty to animals, arson, chambers of horrors.	Immature, ran way from home, was abused as a child.	Poor social relationships.	Bestiality, sadistic killing, knifing, strangulation, criminal confession.

C Starkweather	Animals, guns	Was bullied, immature, school experience, very upsetting to him.	Timid withdrawn.	Multiple killer, spoke in monologues.
F West	Carpentry.	Was bullied at school.	Loner, controlling.	Killing, preservation of sameness.
T McVeigh	Catalogues, animals, mechanics, Start Trek, data reading.	Accident prone, hyperactive, high pain threshold.	Controlling, egocentric, cold and calculating.	Wanderer. Mass killer.
J Dahlmer	Fish, bones, insects, dinosaurs, dead animals, great reader, Blade Runner Movie, satanic bible.	Many infections, poor school performance, naïve, immature, awkward walk.	Loner/shy, poor social cop-on.	When caught- confession to many murders, wanderer, abused alcohol, odd, egocentric, he had preservation of sameness, drugged victims, mutilated victims and cannibalism, frottuer, exhibitionistic, necrophilia.
R Green	Cruelty to animals, arson.	Piercing gaze, was an abused child.	Major social interactional difficulties.	Mutilated victims.
T Wainewright	Art, living beyond his means, great reader, animals.	Naïve and immature, hyperactive.	Callous and unemotional	Poisner for gain.
G Chapman	Criminal matters.	Hyperactive.	Callous and unemotional, egocentric.	Poisoner.
A Chikatilo	Cruelty to animals.	School performance was good enough to lead him to become a school teacher.	Shy, poor social reciprocity.	Knifed victims and gave them slow deaths.
R Berdella	Occult interests, animals, photography of victims, kept meticulous records.		Callous and unemotional.	Experimental killer.
M L Lockhart	Novelty seeking.	Immature.	Egocentric.	Killed for the thrill.
S Matuschka	Engineering.	Immature.	Egocentric.	Wrecked trains to see people suffer.
W Heirens	Medical.	School performance was good enough for him to become a medical student	Shy and unsociable.	Killer, stole women's undergarments.

Table 7. (Continued)

AC Whiteway	Knives, bodybuilding.	In reform school.	Superficial relationships.	Necrophilia.
P Manuel	Great reader, autodictat, art and music.		Controlling.	Housebreaker, killed for the thrill.
Bruno G		Depressed child, high pain threshold.	Loner.	Fearless, fetishism, voyeurism.
JR Christie	Singing, dead bodies, police.		Aloof and reserved.	Strangled victims, necrophilia.
V Connell	Disc jockey, police.		Very controlling	Arson and killing
Case M		"Evil", slow development.		Bestiality, cut up a four year old girl.
Bacher	Cruelty to animals.	"Not normal".	Very poor social relationships.	Killing and mutilating bodies.
V Verzeni	Cruelty to animals.		Silent and solitary.	Heightened sense of smell, sucked blood and relaxed after killing.
Sergeant Bertrand	Cruelty to animals.	Silent child.	Solitary.	Necrophilia.
Ardisson	Stonemason, grave digger.		Solitary, very poor relationship skills.	Necrophilia.
D W	History student.	Immature.	Shy, loner.	Necrophilia.
A Fish	Masochism, sadism.	Immature.		Cannibalism, necrophilia, killing.
MJR Essex	Mechanically minded.	"Good childhood", average in school.		Spree killer.
E Gein	Great reader.	Was bullied.	Very poor social relationships.	Necrophilia, serial killer.
JW Gacy	Children and was a children's entertainer, mathematics.	Very good at jigsaws.	Autistic charisma.	Voyeurism, necrophilia.
A de Salvo		Unsettled childhood, unhappy at school, reform school.	Loner.	Strangler, voyeuristic, criminal confessor.
H Shipman	Letter writing	Average school performance.	Very poor social relationships, egocentric.	Killed over 250 patients.

Glossary

Alexithymia

Persons with Alexithymia tend to be concrete thinkers and have problems describing feelings and emotions.

Algolagnia

This is a phrase used by de River (1951) in discussing sadism with algos meaning pain and lagneia meaning lust.

Amygdala

This is the main area of the brain involved in emotional processing especially of fear, rage, flight, defence, as well as emotional memory. In the brain it is in the shape of an almond.

Androgen

Androgens are substances that produce male characteristics for example testosterone.

Anterior Cingulate Cortex

It helps to determine the emotional salience of stimuli partially when the meaning of the stimuli are unclear. It helps to evaluate past memories in the context of incoming stimuli and allows us to make a decision on incoming stimuli.

Antisocial Personality Disorder

They engage in unlawful behaviour, are deceitful, impulsive, irritable, reckless, irresponsible, and lack remorse.

Asperger's Syndrome

Formally called Autistic Psychopathy. It is not possible to clearly separate from High Functioning Autism. Persons with Asperger's syndrome want to make human contact but have problems with social know-how. While people with High Functioning Autism are very little interested in making human contact. They all show social interactional problems, problems with peer relationships, problems in social and emotional reciprocity. They often avoid eye contact, have problems reading non-verbal behaviour, have narrow interests, preservation of sameness, and show larger problems e.g. pragmatic problems. There is an error in the American Psychiatric Association Classification of Asperger's syndrome which requires no clinically significant general delay in language and no clinically significant delay in language development.

Autonomic Nervous System

This is a nervous system which has two parts – the sympathetic system which increases heart rate, fearfulness and orgasm. The parasympathetic system reduces heart rate and increases intestinal activity common of other activities. These systems function automatically.

Borderline Personality Disorder

These persons show unstable interpersonal relationships, identity disturbance, impulsivity, inappropriate intense anger, long term feelings of emptiness and mood fluctuation.

Cerebellum

It is located at the back of a person's head. It is involved in monitoring movement. It is also involved in thinking for example – cognitive processing of mathematics and involved in social skills as well as language.

Cerebral Cortex

This is an area of the brain that is most highly developed in man and is where the higher cerebral functions take place. It is the outer layer of the brain. Parts of the brain below the cerebral cortex are called subcortical.

Cognitive Processing

This refers to how the mind processes thinking, feeling, etc..

Computerised Tomography (CT)

Allows the imager to examine the structure of the brain.

Corpus Callosum

The nerve fibres of the corpus callosum connect the left and right brain.

Cortisol

This is a hormone associated with stressful situations that a person finds themselves in.

Criminal Autistic Psychopathy

This phrase refers to a resurrection of the concept of Autistic Psychopathy(non-verbal Asperger's syndrome) but associated with criminality. It is basically criminality and autism.

Developmental Disorders

Autism and Asperger's syndrome are developmental disorders, which are disorders with major genetic implications and disordered development.

Dopamine

Is a neurotransmitter that is involved in emotional processing. It is a neurochemical involved in reward. It is involved in sexual interest and sexual interactions.

Dyspraxia

This is associated with clumsiness and motor coordination problems.

Executive Function

This is spoken about when one is discussing the controlling, planning, etc. activities of the frontal lobe.

Foetal Alcohol Syndrome (FAS)

Is associated with substantial intake during pregnancy and is characterised by low birth weight, Hyperkinetic behaviour, wide set eyes, and learning disabilities.

Functional Magnetic Resonance (fMR)

It allows the structure of the brain to be examined from multiple perspectives.

Fusiform Face Area

This is an area of the brain particularly involved in face recognition.

Gamma-aminobutyric Acid (GABA)

GABA is an inhibitory neurotransmitter. Valium increases GABA ergic tone and reduces anxiety.

General Psychopathy

Persons with this are interpersonally exploitative, lack guilt, shame or remorse, are emotionally callous, ruthless, and can be dangerous, have very poor capacity for empathy, can be very dangerous and recidivistic criminals, show a failure to learn from past experiences, and are often cold and indifferent to people.

Grey Matter

Grey cells bodies in the brain as seen under microscopic examination.

Hardwired

This refers to cerebral activity that is genetically underpinned.

Hippocampus

This is a brain structure in the shape of a seahorse. Damage to it leads to problems with learning and retrieving of memories. It is also involved in spatial navigation.

Homovanillic Acid (HVA)

This is a metabolite of Dopamine.

Hypothalamus

The brain structure is involved in regulating appetites and drives.

Insula

It is involved in taste and pain processing as well as emotional processing.

Limbic System

This has a number of parts of the brain associated with it including hippocampal formation, amygdala, hypothalamus and olfactory regions. It is involved with emotional processing, memory and various appetites. It is associated with the emotional brain.

Lutenizing Hormone

It is hypothesized to stimulate libido or sexual interest.

Mentalising

This is the intuitive attribution of mental states for example desires and beliefs to the person themselves and other persons.

Minicolumns

Smallest brain modules for processing information.

Mirror Neurons

Nerve cells active during interpersonal imitation.

Monamine Oxidase (MAO)

It breaks down the amino acid tyramine. It metabolises neurochemicals Dopamine, Serotonin and Noradrenaline.

Narcissistic Personality Disorder

These persons are narcissistic and grandiose, lack empathy, are arrogant, and envious and want to be treated as unique. They tend to exploit people.

Necrophilia

Sexual attraction to corpses.

Neurotransmitter

These are neurochemicals like Serotonin and Dopamine which allow the space between nerve cells and synapse to connect with each other.

Noradrenaline

This is a neurochemical which is associated with the sympathetic nervous system. It is involved in cognitive processing and mood.

Nucleus Accumbens

(Its alternative name is the ventral striatum). It is involved in emotional regulation. It is also involved in reward and pleasure.

Paranoid Personality Disorder

These people are very suspicious, reluctant to confide in other people, bears grudges, and felt that people are doing or saying things to attack them without sufficient reason.

Parietal Lobes

They are involved in spatial processing and the processing of touch and imagery.

Pervasive Developmental Disorders

This is an overarching category from the American Psychiatric Association Classification of Mental Disorders and includes Autistic Disorder, Retts Disorder, Childhood Disintegrative Disorders, Asperger's Disorder, and Pervasive Developmental Disorder Not Otherwise Specified including Atypical Autism. This book is concerned with Autism and Asperger's syndrome and the new category Criminal Autistic Psychopathy.

Positron Emission Tomography (PET)

This is a functional imaging technique which allows the imager to focus on thinking and feeling in the persons brain.

Prefrontal Cortex

This is the executive, managing, controlling area of the brain. It is involved in reflective thought, empathy, and has our sense of self or identity and conscience. It is involved in problem solving and emotional processing. It helps to suppress inappropriate impulses. It is involved in set shifting or shifting from one task to another. It is involved in mentalising that is the attribution of thoughts and feelings to other people as well as to self. It covers an area of about 40% of the total cerebral cortex.

Primary Psychopathy

Persons with this are fearless, callous, organise their criminal activities, have very poor empathy, have very significant genetic factors in aetiology, are often criminal novelty seekers, don't learn from experience and have problems understanding emotional experience.

Schizoid Personality Disorder

Persons with this diagnosis are solitary, lack close friends, show emotional coldness, detachment or evidence flattened feeling states.

Schizotypal Personality Disorder

Persons with this disorder have odd beliefs, odd thinking and speech, are rather paranoid and suspicious, lack close friends, and often show odd behaviour.

Secondary Psychopathy

It has a greater environmental component to the aetiology of psychopathy. There is less planning of psychopathic activities and there is more reactivity. They show somewhat more emotional responsivity than Primary Psychopathy and are a less severe form of disorder. They are more likely to come from deprived damaging environments.

Serotonin

Serotonin is a neurochemical substance in the brain involved at synapses that is connections between cells in the brain. It is a modulator neurotransmitter. Selective Serotonin Reuptake Inhibitors like Prozac block the re-uptake of Serotonin at the synapses. This increases Serotonin there and reduces depression and indeed often anxiety and can calm the brain and increase self-esteem as well. These neurotransmitters help nerve cells to communicate with each other.

Single Photon Emission Computed Tomography (SPECT)

SPECT uses tracers in the blood that follow blood flow and allows the imager to examine the functioning of the brain e.g. thinking, etc..

Social Brain

This refers to the neural networks of nerve cells that underpin our social interactions.

Sociopathy

This is a term that was used particularly in the past when society was blamed for psychopathy. Persons with sociopathy show selfish, callous, irresponsible behaviour who do not learn from experiences.

Synapses

This is the space between nerve cells that allows neurotransmitters which are neurochemical substances in the brain, to make connections that communicates information from one nerve cell to the next.

Temporal Lobes

The temporal lobes are involved in the processing of sensory stimuli e.g. visual stimuli which are then processed. They are also involved in language processing.

Thalamus

It is involved in relayed impulses from various parts of the cortex and subcortical areas.

Theory of Mind / Mind Reading

This involves attributing feelings and desires to other people. It is a decentred perspective.

Vasopressin

Hormone involved in social bonding particularly in monogamous priari voles. In the future it may be shown to be relevant to psychopathy.

Von Econom Neurons

Nerve cells in the brain involved in rapid intuitive decision making.

Weak Central Coherence

This refers to a person's ability to process details very accurately but at the same time being poor at processing the big picture.

White Matter

The colour of the myelin sheets of the fibres emanating from the neuronal body as seen under microscopic examination. These nerve fibres connect different parts of the brain.

REFERENCES

Abel, G. G., Blanchard, E. B. (1974). The Role of Fantasy and the Treatment of Sexual Deviation. *Archives of General Psychiatry*, 30: 467 – 475.

Abell, F., Hare, D. J. (2005). An experimental investigation of the phenomenology of delusional beliefs in people with Asperger's syndrome. *Autism*, 9, 5, 515 – 531.

Adam, H. L. (1930). Trial of George Chapman. William Hodge and Company, Edinburgh.

Alexander, G. E., Crutcher, M. D., De Long, M. R. (1990). Basal ganglia thalamocortical circuits: Parallel substriates for motor, oculomotor, prefrontal and limbic functions. *Progress in Brain Research*, 85, 119 – 146.

Allen, D., Evans, C., Hider, A., Peckett, H. (2006). Asperger's syndrome and Offending Behaviour. Autism Cymru, 2nd International Conference, Cardiff, May 10th 2006.

Allman, J. M. et al. (2001). The anterior cingulated cortex – the evolution of an inter phase between emotion and cognition. *Ann M. Y. Acad., Sci.*, 935, 107 – 117.

Allman, J., Watson, K., Tetreault, N., Hakeem, A. (2005). Intuition and Autism: A Possible Role for Von Economo Neurons, *Trends in Cognitive Sciences*, 9, 8, 367 – 373.

America Law Institute Test Section Four. 01 of the Mental Model Penal Code, Page 167.

American Psychiatric Association (1968). Diagnostic and Statistical Manual of Mental Disorders, 2nd edition, Washington DC: American Psychiatric Association.

American Psychiatric Association (1980). Diagnostic and Statistical Manual of Mental Disorders, 3rd edition, Washington DC: American Psychiatric Association.

American Psychiatric Association (1982). Statement on the Insanity Defence, December 1982.

American Psychiatric Association (1994). Diagnostic and Statistical Manual of Mental Disorders (4th Edition), Washington DC: American Psychiatric Association.

American Psychiatric Association (2000). Diagnostic and Statistical Manual of Mental Disorders (4th Edition), Washington DC: American Psychiatric Association.

Anderson, G., Hoshino, Y. (2005). Chapter 17: Neurochemical studies of Autism. Handbook of Autism and Pervasive Developmental Disorder. Edited by Volkmar F., Paul R., Klin A., Cohen D. J. (2005). John Wiley & Sons.

Andreasen, N. (2004). Brave New Brain. Oxford University Press, 2001. First issued as an Oxford University Press Paperback in 2004.

Asperger, H. (1944/1991). Die "Autistischen Psychopathen" i.m Kindesalter, Archives fur Psychiatrie und Nervenkrankheiten, vol. 117, 76 – 136. Translated in U. Frith (ed.)

Autism and Asperger's syndrome, Cambridge: Cambridge University Press, 1991, pp. 37 – 92.

Asperger, H. (1974). Formen des Autismus bei Kindern, Deutsches Arzteblatt, Vol. 14, 4.

Asperger, H. (1979). Problems of infantile autism, *Communication*, Vol. 13, 45 – 52.

Bailey, A., Lutherd, P., Dean, A. (1998). A Clinicopathological Study of Autism. *Brain*, 121, 889 – 905.

Bailey, S. (1997). Sadistic and violent acts in the young. *Child Psychology and Psychiatry Review*, 2, 3, 92 – 102.

Baron Cohen, S., Knickmeyer, R., Belmont, M. (2005). *Science*, Volume 310, 4th November, Page 819 – 823.

Baron-Cohen, S. (1988). An assessment of violence in a young man with Asperger's syndrome. *British Journal of Psychiatry*, 29, 351 – 360.

Baron-Cohen, S. (2005). Chapter 18: The Empathising System. In Origins of the Social Mind by B. Ellis, D. Bjorklund (Ed) (2005). Guildford Press.

Baron Cohen, S., Knickmeyer, R., Belmont, M. (2005). Sex Differences in the Brain: Implications for Explaining Autism. *Science*, Volume 310, 4th November, Page 819 – 823.

Barry, C. T., Frick, P. J., De Shazo, T. M., McCoy, M. G., Ellis, M., Looney, B. R. (2000). The importance of callous-unemotional traits for extending the concept of psychopathy to children. *Journal of Abnormal Psychology*, 109, 335 – 340.

Barry-Walsh, J. B., Mullen, P. E. (2004). Forensic aspects of Asperger's syndrome. *Journal of Forensic Psychiatry and Psychology*, 15, 1, 96 – 107.

Bartholomew, A., Milte, K., Galbally, F. (1978). *Homosexual Necrophilia Med. Sci. Law*, 18, 1, 29 – 35.

Bassarath, C. (2001). Neuroimaging studies of antisocial behaviour. *Canadian Journal of Psychiatry*, Volume 46, Page 728 – 732.

Bataille, G. (1965). Le proces de Gilles de Rais. Paris. Jean-Jacques Pauvert.

Baumeister, R. F. (1997). Evil: Inside Human Cruelty and Violence. W. H. Freeman & Company, New York.

Beitman, B., Nair, J. (2004). Self Awareness Deficits in Psychiatric Patients: Neurobiology, Assessment, and Treatment. W. W. Norton & Company, New York.

Beitman, B., Nair, J., Viamontes, G. Chapter 1: Why self-awareness? In Self Awareness Deficits in Psychiatric Patients: Neurobiology, Assessment, and Treatment. Edited by B. Beitman and J. Nair. W. W. Norton & Company, New York: 2004.

Berg, C. (1938). The Sadist. Translated by O. Illner and G. Godwin. Published by Acorn Press London.

Bettelheim, B. (1967). The Empty Fortress: Infantile Autism and the Birth of the Self. Published by the Free Press, New York.

Bishop, S., Lam, M., Devins, G. (2004). Mindfulness: A proposed Operational Definition. Clinical Psychology: *Science and Practice*, vii N3 Fall, 230 – 240.

Blackburn, R. (1988). On moral judgement and personality disorders. The myth of the psychopathic personality revisited. *British Journal of Psychiatry*, 153, 505 – 512.

Blackburn, R. (1996). Psychopathy and Personality Disorder: Implications of Interpersonal Theory. Issues in *Criminological and Legal Psychology*, 24, 18 – 23.

Blackburn, R. (2006). Chapter 3: Other Theoretical Models of Psychopathy. Chapter in Handbook of Psychopathy, Edited by C. J. Patrick, Guildford Press, New York, 2006.

Blackman, L. (2001). Lucy's story: Autism and other adventures. London: Jessica Kingsley Publishers.

Blair, J. R., Cipolotti, L. (2000). Impaired social response reversal: A case of acquired sociopathy. *Brain*, 123, 1122 – 1141.

Blair, J., Mitchell, D., Blair, K. (2005). The Psychopath. Blackwell: Oxford.

Blair, J., Sellars, C., Strickland, I., Clarke, F., Williams, A., Smith, A., Jones, L. (1996). Theory of mind in psychopaths. *Journal of Forensic Psychiatry*, 7, 1, 15 – 25.

Blair, R. J. (1995). A cognitive developmental approach to morality: Investigating the psychopath. *Cognition*, 57, 1 – 29.

Blair, R. J. Chapter 15: Subcortical Brain Systems in Psychopathy: The Amygdala and Associated Structures. Page 296 – 313. Chapter in Handbook of Psychopathy, Edited by C. J. Patrick, Guildford Press, New York, 2006.

Blair, R. J. R., Budhani, S., Colledge, D., Scott, S. (2005). Deafness to fear in boys with psychopathic tendencies. *Journal of Child Psychology Psychiatry*, 46, 3, 327 – 336.

Blair, R. J., Frith, U. (2000). Neurocognitive explanations of Antisocial Personality Disorder. *Criminal Behaviour and Mental Health*, 10, 566 – 582.

Blair, R. J., Mitchell, D. G., Richell, R. A., Kelly, S., Leonard, H., Newman, C., Scott, S. (2002). Turning a deaf ear to fear: Impaired recognition of vocal affect in psychopathic individuals. *Journal of Abnormal Psychology*, 11, 682 – 686.

Blair, R. J., Peschardt, K. S., Budhani, S., Mitchell, D., Pine, D. S. (2006). The Development of Psychopathy. *Journal Child Psychology Psychiatry*, 47, 3 / 4, 262 – 275.

Blakemore, C. (1988). The Mind Machine. BBC Books: London.

Blum, D. (1997). Sex on the Brain. Viking Penguin.

Bogdashina, O. (2005). Sensory issues in autism are recognised. http//www.awares.org-conferences.

Bosch, G. (1970). Infantile autism. Translated by D. Jordan and I. Jordan. New York: Springer-Verlag.

Boss, M. (1949). Meaning and Content of Sexual Perversions, New York: Grune and Stratton.

Bremner, M. (1991). Republication of Juliette by de Sade. The Times, Tuesday October 13th 1991.

Brittain, R. P. (1970). The Sadistic Murderer. *Medical Science and the Law*, 10, 198 – 207.

Britton, P. (1995). Fred West. They Grew Into Monsters. Sunday Times New Review, 26, Page 1 – 2.

Browne, W. A. F. (1875). Necrophilism. *Journal of Mental Science*, 20, 551.

Bruch, H. (1967). Mass Murder: The Wagner Case. *American Journal of Psychiatry*, 124: 5, Page 147, 693 – 698.

Burgess, A. W., Hartman, C. R., Ressler, R. R. (1986). Sexual Homicide: A Motivational Model. *Journal of Interpersonal Violence*, 1: 251 – 252.

Cahill, L. (2005). His brain, her brain. Scientific American, May, 22 – 29.

Camus, A. (1946). The Outsider. (Eng. Trans). (L'Estranger, 1942).

Casanova, M. (2005). Abnormalities in Brain Circuitry in Autism. http//www.awares.org-conferences.

Cawthorne, N. (2002). The Worlds Greatest Serial Killers. Chancellor Press: London.

Chalidze, V. (1977). Criminal Russia by. Published by Random House, New York.

Churchland, P. (1998). Towards the Cognitive Neurobiology of the Moral Virtues. *Topoi*. 17: 83 – 86.

Churchland, P. (2005). Brain Based Values, American Scientist, Volume 93, Page 356 – 358.

Clare, A. (1999). Dangerous Liaisons. Sunday Times Books, 1st August, Page 8 – 9.

Clekley, H. (1950). The Mask of Sanity. St. Louis, MO: Mosby.

Clekley, H. (1976). The Mask of Sanity, 5th Edition, St. Louis W. O.

Clekley, H. C. (1941). The Mask of Sanity: An attempt to reinterpret the so-called Psychopathic Personality. St. Louis MO: Mosby (4th Edition, 1967).

Cloninger, C. R. (1987). A systematic method for clinical description and classification of personality variance. *Archives of General Psychiatry*, 44, 573 – 588.

Cloninger, C. R., Svarkic, D. M., Pryzbeck, T. R. (1993). A psychobiological model of temperament and character. *Archives of General Psychiatry*, 34: 136 – 145.

Cohen, D., Strayer, J. (1996). Empathy and conduct disorders and comparison youth. *Developmental Psychology*, 32, 988 – 999.

Committee on Substance Abuse and Committee on Children with Disabilities, (1993). Foetal Alcohol Syndrome and Foetal Alcohol Affects. *Paediatrics*, 91: 1004 – 1006.

Conradi, P. (1992). The Red Ripper. True Crime: London.

Cooke, D. J., Michie, C. (2001). Refining the construct of psychopathy: Towards a hierarchical model. *Psychological Assessment*, 13, 2, 171 – 188.

Cooke, D., Michie, C., Hart, S., Clarke, C. (2005). Assessing psychopathy in the U.K. *British Journal of Psychiatry*, 186, 335 – 341.

Corvin, (1952). In Haire N. Sexual Anomalies and Perversions. Encyclopaedic Press: London.

Coward, D. (1991). Pornocrat or Libertarian? The Moral Darwinism of De Sade. Times Literary Supplement, February 15th 1991, Page 5.

Coward, D. (2005). Review of How to Read Sade. Times Literary Supplement, April 22nd Page 26.

Craig, A. D. (2004). Human Feelings: Why Are Some More Aware than Others? *Trends in Cognitive Sciences*, 8, 6, 239 – 241.

Craig, J., Hatton, C., Craig, F., Bentall, R. (2004). Persecutory beliefs, attributions and theory of mind: Comparison of patients with paranoid delusions, Asperger's syndrome, and healthy controls. *Schizophrenia Research*, 69, 29 – 33.

Dahlmer, L. (1995). A Father's Story. Published by Warner Books. London.

Daly, M., Wilson, M. (1988). Homicide New York: Aldine de Druyter.

Damasio, A. R. (1994). Descartes error: Emotion reason and the human brain. New York: Picador.

Davenport-Hines, R. (2001). Marquis De Sade. Doing Some Measuring Ahead of Time. London Review of Books, 9th August, 15 – 16.

Davison J. (1983) Oswald's Game Norton: New York

De River, J. P. (1956). The Sexual Criminal. Charles C. Thomas: Springfield.

De Slincourt, A. (Trans) (1972). Herodotus: The Histories: Penguin. Harmondsworth.

De Wied, M., Goudena, P., Matthys, W. (2005). Empathy in boys with disruptive behaviour disorders. *Journal of Child Psychology Psychiatry*, 46, 8, 867 – 880.

Debbaudt, D. (2002). Autism Advocates and Law Enforcement Professionals: Recognising and reducing risk situations for people with Autism Spectrum Disorder. London / Philadelphia, Jessica Kingsley Publishers.

Debbaudt, D. (2003). Safety issues for adolescents with Asperger's syndrome. In L. H. Willey (Ed) Asperger's syndrome in Adolescents. Living with the ups, the downs, and things in between. London: Jessica Kingsley Publishers.

Debbaudt, D. (2004). Are you prepared for an autism emergency? Denis Debbaudt's Autism Risk and Safety Newsletter. Port St. Lucia, Florida.

Debbaudt, D., Coles, D. (2004). The role of the family / school liaison counsellor: Safety and risk support for students with Autism Spectrum Disorder. Autism Spectrum Quarterly.

Depue, R. L., Schindehette, S. (2005). From Between Good and Evil. Warner Books: New York.

Dick, P. K. (1982). Do Androids Dream of Electric Sheep. (Originally published in 1973). New York: Ballantine Books. Deeley M. (Producer) and Scott R. (Director). (1982).

Dietz, P. E. (1986). Mass, Serial, and Sensational Homicides. Bulletin N. Y.: *Acad. Med.*, 62, 477 – 91.

Dobbs, D. (2006). Mastery of Emotions. Scientific American Mind, February / March 2006, Page 44 – 49, Volume 17, No. 1.

Dolan, B., Coid, J. (1993). Psychopathic and Antisocial Personality Disorders. Gaskell: London.

Dolan, M. (2004). Neurological factors in aggressive children and adults. In S. Bailey and M. Dolan. *Adolescent Forensic Psychiatry*. Arnold: London.

Dolan, M., Millington, J. (2004). Chapter 9: Personality Dysfunction and Disorders in Childhood and Adolescence, Page 115 – 121. In S. Bailey and M. Dolan (Eds), 2004, *Adolescent Forensic Psychiatry*, Arnold: London.

Domschke, K., Sheehan, K., Lowe, L., Kirley, A., Mullins, C., O'Sullivan, R., Freitage, C., Becker, T., Conroy, J., Fitzgerald, M., Gill, M., Hawi, Z. (2005). Association analysis of the Monamine Oxidase A & B genes with Attention Deficit Hyperactivity Disorder in an Irish sample: Preferential transmission of the MAO-A 941G allele to affected children. *American Journal of Medical Genetics*, 134, 1, 110 – 114.

Dostoevsky, F. (1980). The Brothers Karamazov. Taken from L. Wolf, 1980, Bluebeard. The Life and Times of Gilles de Rais.

Dostoevsky, F. Stavrogin's Confession, Page 43. Taken from L. Wolf, 1980, Bluebeard. The Life and Times of Gilles de Rais.

Douglas Fields, R. (2005). Erasing memories. Scientific American Mind, November, 29 – 35.

Du Plessix Gray, F. (1999). At Home with the Marquis de Sade. Chatto and Windus, London.

Eisenberg, N. (2000). Emotion, regulation, and moral development. *Annual Review of Psychology*, 51, 665 – 697.

Ellis, H. D., Ellis, D., Fraser, W., Deb, S. (1994). A preliminary study of right hemisphere cognitive deficits and impaired social judgements among young people with Asperger's syndrome. *European Child & Adolescent Psychiatry*, 3, 4, 255 – 266.

Emsley, J. (2005). Elements of Murder. Oxford University Press.

Everall, I., Le Couter, A. (1990). Fire setting in an adolescent boy with Asperger's syndrome. *British Journal of Psychiatry*, 157, 284 – 287.

Fenigstein, A., Venable, P. A. (1992). Paranoid and self conscious. *J. Person. And Soc. Psychology*, 62, 129 – 134.

Fido, M. (2001). A History of British Serial Killing. Carlton: London.

Fitzgerald, M. (2001). Autistic Psychopathy. *Journal of the American Academy of Child and Adolescent Psychiatry*, 40, 8, 870.

Fitzgerald, M. (2001). Borderline Psychopathology. *Journal of the American Academy of Child and Adolescent Psychiatry*, 40, 10, 1124.

Fitzgerald, M. (2003). Callous-unemotional traits and Asperger's syndrome. *Journal of the American Academy of Child and Adolescent Psychiatry*, 42, 9, 1011.

Fitzgerald, M. (2004). Autism and Creativity. Brunner Routledge Hove.

Fitzgerald, M. (2004). Features of Alexithymia or features of Asperger's syndrome. *European Child and Adolescent Psychiatry*, 13, 2, 123.

Fitzgerald, M. (2005). Borderline Personality Disorder and Asperger's syndrome. *Autism*, 9, 4, 452.

Fitzgerald, M. (2005). Malignant alienation or Asperger's syndrome. *Journal of Psychiatric Practice*, 29, 5, 193.

Fitzgerald, M. (2005). The Genesis of Artistic Creativity. London: Jessica Kingsley.

Fitzgerald, M., Bellgrove, M. (2006). The overlap between Alexithymia and Asperger's syndrome. *Journal of Autism and Developmental Disorders*, 36, 4, 573 – 576.

Fitzgerald, M., Corvin, A. (2001). Diagnosis and differential diagnosis of Asperger's syndrome, *Advances in Psychiatric Treatment*, vol. 7, 310 – 318.

Fitzgerald, M., Gallagher, L. (In Press). Overlap of Attention Deficit Hyperactivity Disorder and Asperger's syndrome. In Fitzgerald M., Bellgrove M., Gill M. Handbook of Attention Deficit Hyperactivity Disorder. In Press. Wiley.

Fombonne, E. (2005). Epidemiological studies of Pervasive Developmental Disorders. In Handbook of Autism and Pervasive Developmental Disorder. Edited by Volkmar F., Paul R., Klin A., Cohen D. J. (2005). John Wiley & Sons.

Fonagy, P. (2003). Towards a developmental understanding of violence. *British Journal of psychiatry*, 183, 190 – 192.

Fowles, D. C., Dindo, L. (2006). Chapter 2: A dual-deficit model of psychopathy. Chapter in Handbook of Psychopathy, Edited by C. J. Patrick, Guildford Press, New York, 2006.

France, J. (1998). Communication Speech and Language in the Forensic Psychotherapy in Forensic Psychotherapy edited by C. Cordess and M. Cox. Jessica Kingsley.

Frank, G. (1967). The Boston Strangler. Published by Jonathan Cape. London.

Franke, D. (1975) The Torture Doctor. Published by Hawthorn Books, New York.

Frick, P., Marsee, M. (2006). Chapter 18: Psychopathy and Developmental Pathways to Antisocial Behaviour in Youth, Page 353 – 374. Chapter in Handbook of Psychopathy, Edited by C. J. Patrick, Guildford Press, New York, 2006.

Frith, U. (1991). (Ed.) Autism and Asperger's syndrome, Cambridge: Cambridge University Press.

Gaddis, T. (1985). Birdman of Alcatraz. London: Gollanz.

Gaddis, T. E., Long, J. O. (1970). Killer: A Journal of Murder, New York: MacMillan.

Gallwey, P. L. G. (1985). The psychodynamics of Borderline Personality in D. Farrington and J. Gunn (Eds.) Aggression and Dangerousness. New York: Wiley, 127 – 152.

Gazzaniga, M., Steven, M. (2005). *Neuroscience and the Law*, 16, 1, Page 43 – 49.

Gerrard, N. (1995). The West's. Rosemary's Babies. Sunday, November 26th, The Review (Observer), Page 1.

Geurts, H. M., Verte, S., Wosterlaan, J., Royers, H., Sergeant, J. A. (2004). How Specific are Executive Function Deficits in Attention Deficit Hyperactivity Disorder and Autism? *Journal of Child Psychology and Psychiatry*, 45, 4, 836 – 854.

Ghaziuddin, M., Tsai, L., Ghaziuddin, N. (1991). Brief Report: Violence in Asperger's syndrome, a critique. *Journal of Autism and Developmental Disorders*, 21, 3, Page 349 – 354.

Ghaziuddin, M., Tsai, L., Ghaziuddin, N. (1991). Brief Report: Violence in Asperger's syndrome, a critique. *Journal of Autism and Developmental Disorders*, 22, 4, 643 – 649.

Gillberg, C. (1991). Clinical and neurobiological aspects of Asperger's syndrome. In U. Frith (ed.) Autism and Asperger's syndrome, Cambridge: Cambridge University Press, p. 123.

Gillberg, C. (1995). Clinical child neuropsychiatry. Cambridge University Press: Cambridge.

Gillberg, C. (1996). Book Review. Loners by S. Wolff. *European Child & Adolescent Psychiatry*, 5, 178.

Gillberg, C. (2002). A guide to Asperger's syndrome. Cambridge University Press: Cambridge.

Gillberg, C., Coleman, M. (2000). The biology of autistic syndromes. MacKeith Press: London.

Goldberg, E. (2001). The Executive Brain: Frontal Lobes and the Civilised Mind.

Goldhagen, D. J. (1997). Hitler's Willing Executioners, Abacus: London.

Golding, W. (1954). Lord of the Flies.

Goya, F. Preface Two, Lost Caprichos, quoted by Anthony Storr (1992) in Human Destructiveness. Routledge.

Grandin, T. (1996). Thinking in pictures and other reports from my life with autism. New York: Vintage books.

Gregory, R. (Ed.) (2004). The Oxford Companion to the Mind. Oxford University Press: Oxford.

Grewal, D., Salovey, P. (2005). Feeling Smart: The Science of Emotional Intelligence. *American Scientist*, Volume 93, Page 330 – 339.

Grubin, D. (1994). Sexual Murder. *British Journal of Psychiatry*, 165, 624 – 629.

Grubin, D. (1997). Predictors of Risk in Serious Sex Offenders. *British Journal of Psychiatry*, 170 (Suppl. 32), 17 – 21.

Gunn, J. (1978). The treatment of psychopaths. In Gaind, R. (ed.) Current Themes in Psychiatry, London: MacMillan.

Gunn, J. (1998). Psychopathy: An elusive concept with moral overtones. In T. Millon et al. (1998). Psychopathy. Gardner Press: New York.

Haire, N. (1952). Sexual Anomalies and Perversions. A summary of the Works of the late Prof. Dr. Magnus Hirschfeld. Encyclopaedic Press: London.

Hansen, H. (1998). Treating the untreatable in Denmark. In Millon T. (1998). 7th Edition, Psychopathy. Gardner Press: New York.

Hansford Johnson, P. (1967). On Iniquity: Some Personal Reflections Arising Out of the Moors Murder Trial. MacMillan: London.

Harbort, S., Mokros, A. (2001). Serial Murderers in Germany from 1945 to 1995. Homicide Studies, Volume 5, No. 4, November 2001, Page 311 – 334.

Hare, R. D. (1970). Psychopathy: Theory and Research. New York: Wiley.

Hare, R. D. (1986). Twenty Years of Experience with the Clekley Psychopath. In W. H. Reid, D. Dorr, J. I. Walker, and G. W. Bonner (Eds). Unmasking the Psychopath: Antisocial Personality and Related Syndromes, New York: Norton.

Hare, R. D. (1991). Manual for the Hare Psychopathy Checklist – Revised. Toronto: Multi-Health Systems.

Hare, R. D., Gould, J., Mills, R., Wing, L. (1999). A preliminary study of individuals with Autism Spectrum Disorders in three special hospital in England. London: National Autistic Society.

Hare, R. D., Jutai, J. W. (1988). Psychopathy and cerebral asymmetry in semantic processing. *Personality and Individual Differences*, 9, 2, 329 – 337.

Harmer, C. J., Bhagwager, Z., Peret, D., Voll, M. B., Cohen, P., Goodwin, G. (2003). Acute SSRI Administration Affects the Processing of Social Cues in Healthy Volunteers. *Neuropsychopharmacology*, 28, 148 – 152.

Harmer, C. J., Rogers, R., Tunbridge, E., Cowen, P., Goodwin, G. (2003). Tryptophan Depletion Increases the Recognition of Fear in Female Volunteers. *Psychopharmacology*, 167, 411 – 417.

Harper, T. J., Hare, R., D., Hakstein, A. R. (1989). Two factor conceptualisation of psychopathy. *Psychological Assessment*, 1, 6 – 17.

Harpur, J., Lawlor, M., Fitzgerald, M. (2004). Succeeding in College with Asperger's syndrome. Published by Jessica Kingsley.

Harpur, J., Lawlor, M., Fitzgerald, M. (2006). Succeeding with Interventions for Asperger's syndrome and Adolescents. London Jessica Kingsley.

Harpur, T. J., Hare, R. D., Hakstian, A. R. (1989). Two-factor conceptualisation of psychopathy: Construct validity and assessment implications. *Journal of Consulting and Clinical Psychology*, 1, 6 – 17.

Harris G., Rice, M. Chapter 28: Treatment of Psychopathy: A Review of Empirical Findings, Page 555 – 572. Chapter in Handbook of Psychopathy, Edited by C. J. Patrick, Guildford Press, New York, 2006.

Haslam, A., Reichter, S. D. (2005). The Psychology of Tyranny, Page 44 – 51. *Scientific American Mind*, 16 3.

Hawkes, N. (1995). Female and Male Brains Differ. The Times, Friday January 27th, Page 7.

Hazelwood, R. R., Warren, J., Dietz, P. E. (1993). Compliant Victims of the Sexual Sadist. *Australian Family Physician*, 1993, 22, 4, Page 474 – 79.

Hazelwood, R., Warren, J. (1995). The prevalence of fantasy in sexual crimes investigation. In Hazelwood R., Burgess A. (Eds). Practical Aspects of Rape Investigation. N. Y.: Elsevier.

Herbert, I., Akbar, D. (2004). The death of Harold Shipman. The Independent, Wednesday 14th of January, Page 6.

Herve, H. F., Hayes, P. J., Hare, R. D. (2003). Psychopathy and Sensitivity to the Emotional Polarity of Metaphorical Statements. *Personality and Individual Differences*, 35, 1497 – 1507.

Hiatt, K., Newman, J. (2006). Chapter 17: Understanding Psychopathy: The Cognitive Side, Page 334 – 352. Chapter in Handbook of Psychopathy, Edited by C. J. Patrick, Guildford Press, New York, 2006.

Hickey, E. (1991). Serial Murderers and Their Victims. Belmont CA: Wadsworth.

Hill, E., Frith, U. (2003). Understanding Autism: Insights from Mind and Brain. *Phil. Trans. Soc. Lond. B.*, 358, 281 – 289.

Hill, J. (2002). Biological, psychological and social processes in Conduct Disorders. *Journal of Child Psychology Psychiatry*, 43, 1, 133 – 164.

Hines, M. (2004). Brain Gender. Oxford University Press.

Hirschfeld, (1952). Sexual Anomalies. Emerson Books, New York.

Hirstein, W., Iversen, P., Ramachandran, V. S. (2001). Autonomic response of autistic children to people and objects. Proc. R. Soc. Lond. B 268, 1883 – 1888.

Hitchings, H. (1999). Sadistic longings. New Statesman, 17th May, Page 46 – 47.

Hobbes, T. (1651). The Leviathan.

Hobson, R. P., Meyer, J. A. (2005). Foundations for Self and Other: Study in Autism. *Developmental Science*, 8, 6, 481 – 491.

Hoffman, M. L. (2000). Empathy and moral development: Implications for and justice. Cambridge University Press: Cambridge.

Holden, A. (1995). The St. Alban's Poisoner. Corgi Books, London.

Holmes, J., Payton, A., Barrett, J., Harrington, R., McGuffin, P., Owen, M., Ollier, W., Worthington, J., Gill, M., Kirley, A., Hawi, Z., Fitzgerald, M., Asherson, P., Curran, S., Mill, J., Gould, A., Taylor, E., Kent, L., Craddock, N., Thapar, A. (2002). Association of DRD4 in children with Attention Deficit Hyperactivity Disorder and comorbid conduct problems. *American Journal of Medical Genetics*, 114, 150 – 153.

Hooke, A. E. (2005). Justice and Biology Revisited. Philosophy Now, January / February, Page 20 – 22.

Howlin, P. (1997). Autism preparing for adulthood. London: Routledge.

Howlin, P. (2000). Outcome in adult life for more able individuals with Autism or Asperger's syndrome. *Autism,* 4, 63 – 83.

Hucker, S. (1990). William Faulkner's Story: A Rose for Emily.

Hucker, S. (1990). Chapter 9: Necrophilia and Other Unusual Philias, Page 723 – 727. In Principals and Practice of Forensic Psychiatry, edited by Robert Bluglass and Pal Bowden and published by Churchill Livingston, Edinburgh, 1990.

Huxley, T. H. (1982). Evolution and ethics. Princeton University Press, Princeton N. J.

Hyman, S. (2002). In: Neuroethics: Mapping the Field. Conference Proceedings, May 13th – 14th 2002, California. The Dana Foundation, 2002, New York.

Jensen, V. K., Larrieu, J. A., Mack, K. (1997). Differential Diagnosis Between Attention Deficit / Hyperactivity Disorder and Pervasive Developmental Disorder Not Otherwise Specified. *Clinical Paediatrics*, 36, 555 – 561.

Jones Robinson, R. G. (2002). The Mammoth Book of Women Who Kill. London.

Kalman, F. J. (1938). The Genetics of Schizophrenia. New York: Locust Valley.

Kanner, L. (1943). Autistic disturbances of affective contact. *Nervous Child*, 2, 217 – 250.

Kanner, L. (1951). The conception of wholes to parts in early infantile autism, *American Journal of Psychiatry*, vol. 108, 23 – 9.

Kanner, L. (1973). Autistic disturbances of affective contact. In Kanner L. (Ed). Childhood psychosis: Initial studies and new insights. Winston. Washington DC.

Kanwisher, N. (2006). What's In a Face? Science, 311, 3rd February 2006, 61 – 62.

Karpmin, B. (1948). The Myth of the Psychopathic Personality. *American Journal of Psychiatry*, 104, 523 – 534.

Kelleher, M. D. Kelleher, C. L.. (1998). Murder Most Rare: The Female Serial Killer. Praeger Westport. Connecticut.

Kemper, T. L., Bauman, M. L. (1998). Neuropathology of infantile autism. *Journal of Neuropathology and Experimental Neurology*, 57, 645 – 652.

Kendell, R. E. (2002). The distinction between personality disorder and mental illness, 180, 110 – 115.

Kerr, M., Tremblay, R. E., Pagani, L. (1997). Boys: Behavioural inhibition and the risk of later delinquency. *Archives of General Psychiatry*, 54, 809 – 816.

Kershaw, I. (1998). Hitler. London: Allen Lane.

Kiehl, K., Smith, A. M., Hare, R. D., Meudrer, A., Forster, B. D., Brunk, J., Liddle, P. F. (2001). Limbic abnormalities in affective processing by criminal psychopaths as revealed by functional magnetic imagery. *Biological Psychiatry*, 50, 677 – 684.

Kirley, A., Lowe, N., Mullins, C., McCarron, M., Daly, G., Walman, I., Fitzgerald, M., Gill, M., Hawi, Z. (2004). Phenotype studies of the DRD4 gene polymorphisms in Attention Deficit Hyperactivity Disorder: Association with Oppositional Defiant Disorder and Positive Family History. *American Journal of Medical Genetics, Part B – Neuropsychiatric Genetics*, 131B, 1, 38 – 42.

Klein, M. Love Guilt and Reparation. Quoted in Symington International Review of Psychoanalysis. Symington N. (1980). Response Aroused by the Psychopath. Internal Review of Psychoanalysis, Volume Seven.

Klin, A., Volkmar, F. R. (1997). Asperger's syndrome. In Handbook of Autism and Pervasive Developmental Disorder. Edited by Volkmar F., Paul R., Klin A., Cohen D. J. (2005). John Wiley & Sons.

Kohn, W., Fahum, T., Ratzoni, G., Apter, A. (1998). *Israel Journal of Psychiatry, Relate Sci*, 35, 4, 293 – 299.

Kozol, E., Boucher, R. J., Garofalo, R. F. (1972). The diagnosis and treatment of dangerousness. *Crime and Delinquency*, 39, 1257 – 1261.

Kraepelin, E. (1909 – 1915). Psychiatrie (8th Edition, Volume 4). Leipzig: J. A. Barth Verlag.

Kraepelin, E. (1968). Lectures on Clinical Psychiatry (T. Johnstone, Trans. and Ed), London: Bailliere.

Kugler, B. (1998). The differentiation between autism and Asperger's syndrome. *Autism*, 2, 1, 11 – 32.

Lalumiere, M. L., Harris, G. T., Rice, M. (2001). Psychopathy and developmental disability. *Evolution and behaviour*, 22, 75 – 92.

Langevin, R. (1991). The Sex Killer. In Burgess A. (Editor). Rape and Sexual Assault, Volume 3, New York: Garland.

Langevin, R., Paitich, D., Russon, A. E. (1985). Are Rapist Sexually Anomalous, Aggressive or Both? In Erotic Preference, Gender Identity, and Aggression in Men: New Research Studies. Edited by Langevin R., Hillsdale N. J., Lawrence Erlbaum Associates.

Laqueur, W. (2005). To Cut a Throat Slowly. Times Literary Supplement, December 9th, Page 3 – 4.

Laucht, M., Becker, K., El-Faddagh, M., Hohm, E., Schmidt, M. (2005). Association of DRD4 Exon III Polymorphism with smoking in 15 year olds: A mediating role for novelty seeking? *Journal of the American Academy of Child and Adolescent Psychiatry*, 44, 5, 477 – 484.

Lauffer, D. (2004). Asperger's syndrome, Empathy and Blade Runner. Blade Runner (Motion Picture). US: Warner Brothers. *Journal of Autism and Developmental Disorders*, 34, 5, 587 – 588.

Le Doux, J. (2002). Synaptic self. MacMillan: London.

Leith, W. (1991). Independent on Sunday, 18th August 1991, Page 23.

Lenzen, M. (2005). Feeling our Emotions. *Scientific American Mind*, 16, 1, Page 14 – 15.

Levin, J., Fox, J. (1985). Mass murder: Americas Growing Menace: New York: Plenum.

Lewis, A. (1953). Health is a social concept. *British Journal of Sociology*, 4, 109 – 124.

Leyton, E. (1986). Hunting Humans: The Rise of the Modern Multiple Murderer. New York: Penguin, Page 331.

Leyton E. (1989). Charles Starkweather. Hunting Humans, Penguin.

Leyton, E. (1989). Hunting Humans. Penguin Books. First published in 1986.

Lindsay, P., Webber, J. Chapter 45: In The Mammoth Book of Women Who Kill. Edited by Richard Glynn Jones Robinson: London: 2002.

Lloyd, R. (2006). Men and women wired to feel emotions differently. Irish Examiner, Saturday 22nd 2006, Page 11.

Looney, D., Butler, M., Lima, E., Count, C., Eckel, L. (2006). *Journal of Child Psychology Psychiatry*, 47, 1, 30 – 36.

Lorenz, A. R., Newman, J. P. (2002). Deficient response modulation and emotional processing in low-anxious Caucasian psychopathic offenders: Results from a Lexical Decision Task Emotion, 2, 2, 91 – 104.

Lord, C., Rutter, M., Le Couteur, A. (1994). Autism Diagnostic Interview – Revised: A revised version of a diagnostic interview for caregivers of individuals with possible developmental disorders. *Journal of autism and Developmental Disorders*, 24, 659 – 685.

Lowe, N., Kirley, A., Mullins, C., Fitzgerald, M., Gill, M., Hawi, Z. (2004). Multiple marker analysis at the promoter region of the DRD4 gene and Attention Deficit Hyperactivity Disorder. Evidence of linkage and association with the SNP-616. *American Journal of Medical Genetics, Part B – Neuropsychiatric Genetics*, 131B, 1, 33 – 37.

Lucas, N. (1974). The Sex Killers. Star Book: W. H. Allan, London.

Lykken, D. D. (1995). The Antisocial Personalities. Hillsdale N. J.: Erlbaum. Has Schindler.

Lykken, D. T. (2006). Chapter 1: Psychopathic Personality: The Scope of the Problem. Chapter in Handbook of Psychopathy, Edited by C. J. Patrick, Guildford Press, New York, 2006.

Lynam, D. R. (1996). The early identification of chronic offenders: Who is the fledgling psychopath? *Psychological Bulletin*, 120, 209 – 234.

Lynam, D. R. (1997). Pursuing the psychopath: Capturing the fledgling psychopath in a nomological net. *Journal of Abnormal Psychology*, 106, 425 – 438.

Lynam, D. R. (1998). Early identification of the fledgling psychopath; locating the psychopathic child in current nomenclature. *Journal of Abnormal Psychology*, 107, 566 – 575.

Lynam, D. R. (2002). Fledging Psychopathy. *Law and Human Behaviour*, 26, 255 – 259.

Lyons, V., Fitzgerald, M. (2004). Humour in Autism and Asperger's syndrome. *Journal of Autism and Developmental Disorders*, 34, 5, 521 – 531.

MacCulloch, M. J., Snowden, P. R., Wood, P. J. W., Mills, H. E. (1983). Sadistic fantasy, sadistic behaviour, and offending. *British Journal of Psychiatry*, 143, 20 – 29.

Mann, T. (1948). Dr. Fastus. New York: Alfred Knopf.

Mann, T. (1959). Last Essays. New York: Alfred Knopf.

Mann, T. Dostoevsky – Within Limits. In Thomas Mann Reader, Ed. Walter Angell, Page 435.

Marsden, C. (2006). Dopamine: The Rewarding Years. *British Journal of Pharmacology*, 147, 136 – 144.

Masters, B. (1993). The Shrine of Jeffrey Dahlmer. Hodden & Stoughton: London.

Masters, R. E. L., Lea, A. Elizabeth Countess Balthory: Countess Dracula.

Mawson, D. (1983). "Psychopaths" in special hospitals. *Psychiatric Bulletin*, 7, 178 – 181.

Mawson, D. C., Grounds, R. J., Tantum, D. (1985). Violence and Asperger's syndrome. *British Journal of Psychiatry*, 147, 566 – 569.

Mayer-Gross, W., Slater, E., Roth, M. (1960). Clinical Psychiatry. Slater E., Roth M. (Eds). Balliere, Tindall, and Cassell: London.

McCarthy, P., Fitzgerald, M., Smith, M. (1984). Prevalence of childhood autism in Ireland. *Irish Medical Journal*, 77, 5, 129 – 130.

McDonald, A., Iacono, W. (2006). Chapter 19: Towards an Integrated Perspective on the Aetiology of Psychopathy, Page 375 – 285.

McGuffin, P., Owen, M., Gottesman, I. (Eds.) (2002). Psychiatric genetics and genomics. Oxford University Press.

McNally, R. T. (1983). Dracula was a woman. McGraw-Hill Books: New York.

Mealey, L. (1995). The socio-biology of psychopathy. *Behaviour and Brain Sciences*, 18, 523 – 599.

Meloy, J. R., Gacono, C. B. (1998). The internal world of the psychopath. In T. Millon (1998). Psychopaths. Gardner Press: New York.

Mesibov, G. B., Shea, V., Adams, L. W. (2001). Understanding Asperger's syndrome and High Functioning Autism. N. Y.: Kluwer Academic: Plenum Press.

Michel, L. Herbeck, D. (2002) American Terrorist. Published by Regan Books, New York.

Miller, G. (2005). Reflecting Another's Mind. *Science*, 308, 12th May, 945 – 947.

Miller, J. G. (1991). Last one over the wall. Columbus OH: Ohio State University Press.

Millon, T., Davis, R. (1998). In psychopaths. Gardner Press: New York.

Millon, T., Davis, R., Millon, C., Escovar, L., Meagher, S. (2000). Personality Disorders in Modern Life. Wiley: New York.

Millon, T., Simonsen, E., Birket-Smith, M., Davis, R. (Eds.). (1998). Psychopathy. Guildford Press: New York.

Minshew, N. J., Sweeney, J. A., Bauman, M. L., Webb, S. J. (2005). Neurologic aspects of autism, Page 473 – 514. Handbook of Autism and Pervasive Developmental Disorder. Edited by Volkmar F., Paul R., Klin A., Cohen D. J. (2005). John Wiley & Sons.

Minzenberg, M., Siever, L. (2006). Chapter 13: Neurochemistry and Pharmacology of Psychopathy and Related Disorders, Page 264. Chapter in Handbook of Psychopathy, Edited by C. J. Patrick, Guildford Press, New York, 2006.

Moir, A., Jessel, D. (1995). A Mind to Crime. Michael Joseph: London.

Motion, A. (2000). Wainewright The Poisoner. Faber and Faber: London.

Morrison, H., Goldberg, H. (2004). My Life Among the Serial Killers. Wiley: Chichester.

Mundy, P. (2003). Annotation: The neural basis of social impairments in autism: The role of the dorsal medial-frontal cortex and anterior cingulate system. *Journal of Child Psychology Psychiatry*, 44, 793 – 809.

Murphy, C. (2004). My Journey into the Mind of the Serial Killer. Irish Independent, 3rd June, Page 2, Page 21.

Murphy, D. G., Critchley, H. D., Schmidt, Z. N. (2002). Asperger's syndrome: A proton magnetic resonance spectroscopy study of brain. *Archives of General Psychiatry*, 59, 885 – 891.

Murphy, J. (1976). Psychiatric labelling in cross-cultural perspective. *Science*, 191, 1019 – 1027.

Murrie, D. C., Warren, J. I., Kristiansson, M., Dietz, P. (2002). Asperger's syndrome and forensic settings. *International Journal of Forensic Mental Health*, 1, 1, 59 – 70.

Nanson, J. L. (1992). Autism in Foetal Alcohol Syndrome: Report of six cases. Alcohol Clin. Exp. Res., 16: 558 – 565.

Nash, J. R. (1975). Blood Letters and Bad Men. Warner Books: New York.

Nash, J. R. (2002). Chapter 21: Irma Grese. In The Mammoth Book of Women Who Kill. Edited by Richard Glynn Jones Robinson: London: 2002.

Nash, J. R. (2002). Chapter 26: Ilse Koch. In The Mammoth Book of Women Who Kill. Edited by Richard Glynn Jones Robinson: London: 2002.

National Autistic Society (United Kingdom) Fact Sheet on Autism. London: National Autistic Society, 2001, 2, Reprint.

Newman, J. P. (1998). Psychopathic behaviour: an information processing perspective. In D. J. Cooke, A. Forth, R. D. Hare (Eds.). Psychopathy: Theory and research and implications for society. Dordrecht: Kluwer.

Nigg, J. (2006) Temperamental and Developmental Psychopathology. *Journal Child Psychology Psychiatry*, 47, 3 / 4, 395 – 422.

O'Brien, G., Bell, G. Chapter 11: Learning Disability, Autism, and Offending Behaviour. Page 144 – 151. In Adolescent Forensic Psychiatry, Edited by S. Bailey, M. Dolan (2004) Arnold.

O'Donnell, B. Chapter 15: Mary Ann Cotton. In The Mammoth Book of Women who Kill. Edited by Richard Glynn Jones Robinson: London: 2002.

O'Donnell, B. Chapter 36: Vera Renzi: Crypt of dead lovers. In The Mammoth Book of Women who Kill. Edited by Richard Glynn Jones Robinson: London: 2002.

O'Keane, V., Moloney, E., O'Neill, H., O'Connor, A. (1992). Blunted prolactin responses to d-fenfluramine in sociopathy. *British Journal of Psychiatry*, 160, 643 – 646.

Oberman, L. Science Daily, 205/04, (http//www.sciencedaily.com.205/04).

Ogden, T. (1989). On the Concept of Autistic – Contiguous Position. *International Journal of Psychoanalysis*, 70, Page 127 – 140.

Olson, H., Streissguth, A., Sampson P., Barr, H., Bookstein, F., Thiede, K. (1997). Association of prenatal alcohol exposure with behavioural and learning problems in adolescents. *Journal of the American Academy of Child and Adolescent Psychiatry*, 36, 9, 1187 – 1194.

Patrick, C. J. (1994). Emotion and psychopathy. *Psychophysiology*, 31, 319 – 330.

Patrick, C. J. (2006). Handbook of Psychopathy. Guildford Press: New York.

Pearse, K., Haist, F., Sedaghat, F. (2004). The brain response to personally familiar faces in autism: Findings of fusiform activity and beyond. *Brain*, 127, 2703 – 2716.

Peters, C. (2005). Harold Shipman. Carlton Books: London.

Phillips, J. (2005). How to Read Sade. Granta Books: London.

Philips, M. L. (2003). Understanding the Neurobiology of Perception. *British Journal of Psychiatry*, 182, 190 – 192.

Pickett, J., London, E. (2005). The Neuropathology of Autism: A Review. *Journal of Neuropathol. Exp. Neurol.* 64, 11, 925 – 935.

Pilgrim, D. (2002). Letter to the Editor, *British Journal of Psychiatry*, 181, 77.

Pinel, P. (1962). Insanity (D. D. Davis, Trans), New York: Haffner (original work published in 1801).

Pinel, P. (1801 / 1977). A treatise on insanity. Bethesda, MD: University Publications of America.
Poe, E. A. The Black Cat in complete work of Edgar Allan Poe.
Porter, S., Woodworth, M. (2006). Chapter 24: Psychopathy and Aggression, Page 481 – 494. Chapter in Handbook of Psychopathy, Edited by C. J. Patrick, Guildford Press, New York, 2006.
Posserud, M. B., Lundenvold, A. J., Gillberg, C. (2006). Autistic features in a total population of 7 – 9 year old children. *Journal of Child Psychology Psychiatry*, 47, 2, 167 – 175.
Prentky, R. (1989). The presumptive role of fantasy in serial sexual homicide. *American Journal of Psychiatry*, 146, 7, 887 – 891.
Prentky, R., Burgess, A., Rokous, F., Ressler, R., Douglas, J. (1989). The Presumptive Role of Fantasy in Serial Sexual Homicide. *American Journal of Psychiatry*, 146: 7, Page 887 – 891.
Raddin, P. (1972). The Trickster, A Study in American Indian Methodology, New York: Schocken Books.
Raine, A. (2002). Annotation: The role of prefrontal deficits, low autonomic arousal, and early child health factors in the development of antisocial and aggressive behaviour in children. *Journal of Child Psychology Psychiatry*, 43, 4, 413 – 434.
Raine, A., Sheard, C., Reynolds, G. P., Lencz, T. (1992). Prefrontal structural and functional deficits associated with individual differences in Schizotypal personality. *Schizophrenia Research*, 7, 237 – 247.
Raine, A., Yang, Y. (2002). Chapter 14: The Neuroanatomical Bases of Psychopathy, Page 278 – 295. Chapter in Handbook of Psychopathy, Edited by C. J. Patrick, Guildford Press, New York, 2006.
Rapin, I., Allen, D. (1983). Developmental language disorder. In Kirk, V. (ed.), Neuropsychology and Language Reading and Spelling, New York: Academic Press, pp. 155–84.
Reinhardt, J. M. (1960). The Murderous Trail of Charles Starkweather. Published by Charles Thomas Publishers Springfield, USA.
Ressler, R., Burgess, A., Douglas, J. (1993). Sexual Homicide. Simon and Schuster: London.
Richards, H. (1998). Evil intent: Violence and disorders of will. In T. Millon et al. (1998). *Psychopathy*,. Gardner Press. New York.
Rogers, L., Ungoed-Thomas, J. (2004). Prison letters reveal Shipman's last crises. Sunday Times, January 18th, Page 12.
Rogers, R. (2005). Chapter 16: The Functional Architecture of the Frontal Lobes: Implications for Research with Psychopathic Offenders. Page 313 – 333. Chapter in Handbook of Psychopathy, Edited by C. J. Patrick, Guildford Press, New York, 2006.
Rossman, J., Resnick, P. (1988). Necrophilia: Analysis of 122 cases involving necrophilic acts and fantasies. *Bulletin of the American Academy of Psychiatry and Law*.
Rossman, J., Resnick, P. (1989). Sexual Attraction to Corpses: A Psychiatric Review of Necrophilia, *Bulletin Acad. Psychiatry, Law*, 17, 2, 153 – 163.
Rourke, B. P. (1988). The syndrome of non-verbal learning disabilities: Developmental manifestations in neurological disease, disorder and dysfunction. *The Clinical Neuropsychologist*, 2, 293 – 330.
Rule, M. (1989). The Stranger Beside Me. Published by Warner Books, New York.

Ryle, A. (1997). The structure and development of Borderline Personality Disorder: A proposed model. *British Journal of Psychiatry*, 170, 82 – 87.
Sacks, O. (1995). An Anthropologist on Mars. Picador: London.
Scadding, J. G. (1967). Diagnosis the clinician and the computer. *Lancet*, ii, 877 – 882.
Schaeffer, N. (1999). Marquis de Sade. Hamish Hamilton: London.
Schmidt, H. (1928). A Hang Man's Diary. Edited by Albrecht Keller.
Schneider, K. (1950). Die pychopatischen Personlichkeiten (9th Edition), Vienna.
Schneider, K. (1958). Psychopathic Personalities (9th Edition, M. Hamilton, trans). London: Cassell (Original Work Published in 1950).
Schneider, M. (1964). La Litterature Fantastique en France Paris: Fayard.
Schore, A. (2003). Affect regulation and disorders of the self. Norton: New York.
Schreiber, F. R. (1983). The Shoemaker. Alan Lane.
Schultz, K., Romanski, E., Tsatsanis, K. (2000). Neurofunctional models of autistic disorders in Asperger's syndrome. In Klin A., Asperger's syndrome. Guildford Press.
Scragg, P., Shah, A. (1994). Prevalence of Asperger's syndrome in a Secure Hospital. *British Journal of Psychiatry*, 165, 679 – 682.
Seaton Wagner, M. (1932). The Monster of Dusseldorf: The Life and Trial of Peter Kurten. London Faber and Faber.
Segal, M. (2005). Can we Cure Fear. *Scientific American Mind*, 1, 45 – 49.
Seto, M., Quinsey, V. Chapter 30: Towards the Future, Page 589 – 601. Chapter in Handbook of Psychopathy, Edited by C. J. Patrick, Guildford Press, New York, 2006.
Semrud-Clickeman, M., Hynd G. W. (1980). Right hemisphere dysfunction in non-verbal learning disability. *Psychological Bulletin*, 107, 196 – 209.
Sereny, G. (2005). Ridiculous assumption that ignores child's needs. The Times, Monday June 13th, p. 20.
Shea, V., Mesibov, G. (2005). Adolescents and adults with Autism. In Handbook of Autism and Pervasive Developmental Disorder. Edited by Volkmar F., Paul R., Klin A., Cohen D. J. (2005). John Wiley & Sons.
Sheridan, M. (2003). Frozen Blood: Serial and Psycho Killers in Ireland. Mentor Books: Dublin.
Siever, L. (1998). Neurobiology in psychopathy. In Millon T., Simonsen E., Birket-Smith M., Davis R. Psychopathy. Guildford press: New York.
Siever, L. J., Amin, F., Coccaro, E. F., Trestman, R. L., Silverman, J. M., Horvath, T. B., Mahon, T. R., Knott, P., Davidson, K. L. (1993). CSF homovanillic acid in Schizotypal personality disorder. *American Journal of Psychiatry*, 150, 1, 149 – 151.
Sigman, M., Capps, L. (1997). Children with autism. Harvard University Press: Cambridge MA.
Simon, R. I. (1996). Bad Men do What Good Men Dream. American Psychiatric Press: Washington DC.
Siponmaa, L., Kristiansson, M., Jonson, C., Nyden, A., Gillberg, C. (2001). Juvenile and young adult mentally disordered offenders: The role of child neuropsychiatric disorders. *Journal of the American Academy of Psychiatry and Law*, 29, 420 – 426.
Skuse, D. H. (2000). *Paediatric Res.*, 47, 9.
Slater, E., Roth, M. (1969). In Clinical Psychiatry. Baillire Tindall and Cassesl: London.
Smith, A. (1759). The theory of moral sentiments. Edited by Raphael D., MacFie A. L. Oxford University Press.

Smith, E. H. Chapter 42: Mrs. Vermilya: The Thrill of the Kill. In The Mammoth Book of Women who Kill. Edited by Richard Glynn Jones Robinson: London: 2002.

Smith, I. (2000). Motor functioning in Asperger's syndrome. In Klin A., Volkmar F., Sparrow S. (2000). Asperger's syndrome. Guildford Press. New York.

Smith, J. (2000). The Guardian, Wednesday September 13th, Page 12 – 13.

Sokol, D. K. (2004). You, your physician and Britain's "Dr. Death". International Herald Tribune, September 13th, Page 8.

Sonderstrom, H. (2003). Psychopathy as a disorder of empathy. *European Child & Adolescent Psychiatry*, 12, 249 – 252.

Sonnenmoser, M. (2005). Friend or foe. *Scientific American Mind*, 78 – 81.

Spitzer, R., Feister, S., Gay, M., Pfohl, E. (1991). Results of a Survey of Forensic Psychiatrists on the Validity of the Sadistic Personality Disorder Diagnosis. *American Journal of Psychiatry*, 148: 7, 1991, Page 875 – 879.

Steinhausen, H. C., Willms, J., Spohr, H. (1993). Long Term Psychopathology and Cognitive Outcome of Children with Foetal Alcohol Syndrome. *Journal of the American Academy of Child and Adolescent Psychiatry*, 32: 990 – 994.

Stone, J. (2002). Autism. Times Literary Supplement, 29th March.

Stone, M. (1998). Sadistic Personality in murderers. In T. Millon. Psychopathy. Gardner Press: New York.

Stone, M. H. (1993). Abnormalities of Personality: Within and Beyond the Realm of Treatment. Norton: New York.

Studholme, B. (2005). In: C. Peters book on Harold Shipman. Carlton Books: London.

Sturup, G. K. (1951). Krogede Skaebner. Copenhagen: Mynksgaard.

Stuss, Chapter 5: The Lost Self. From Self Awareness Deficits in Psychiatric Patients: Neurobiology, Assessment, and Treatment. Edited by B. Beitman and J. Nair. W. W. Norton & Company, New York: 2004.

Sullivan, E., Kosson, D. Chapter 22: Ethnic and Cultural Variations in Psychopathy. Chapter in Handbook of Psychopathy, Edited by C. J. Patrick, Guildford Press, New York, 2006.

Taber, C. W. (1965). Cyclopaedic Medical Dictionary. Oxford: Scientific Publications.

Tancredi, L. (2005). Hardwired Behaviour: What Neuroscience Reveals about Morality. Cambridge University Press.

Tantum, D. (1988). Life long eccentricity and social isolation: Asperger's syndrome or Schizoid Personality Disorder. *British Journal of Psychiatry*, 153: 783.

Tantum, D. (1991). Asperger's syndrome in adulthood. In U. Frith (1991). Autism and Asperger's syndrome. Cambridge University Press: Cambridge.

Tantum, D. (2000). Adolescents and adulthood of individuals with Asperger's syndrome. In Klin A., Volkmar F., Sparrow S. (2000). Asperger's syndrome. Guildford Press: New York.

Teicher, M. (2002). Scars That Wont Heal: The Neurobiology of Child Abuse. *Scientific American*, March 2002, Page 54 – 61.

Thomas, D. (1992). Marquis de Sade. Allison Busby.

Thompson, D. (2005). Review of C. Peters book Harold Shipman. Ireland on Sunday, March 13th, 61.

Thompson, S. (2006). You're Not What you Think. Irish Times, May 2nd, Page 15.

Thorne, M. (2004). Mad, Bad and Dangerous to Know, The Independent, Friday 15th October, Page 29.

Tiihonen, J., Kuikka, J. T. (1997). Single-photo emission tomography imaging of Monamine transporters in impulsive violent behaviour. *Eur J. Nucl. Med.*, 24: 1253 – 1260.

Toal, F., Murphy, D., Murphy, K. (2005). Autistic-Spectrum Disorders: Lessons from neuroimaging. *British Journal of Psychiatry*, 187, 395 – 397.

Trakakis, N. (2004). Interview with William Rowe. Philosophy Now, August September 2004, Page 16 – 17.

Tsai, L. (2001). From autism to Asperger's disorder, American Academy of Child and Adolescent Psychiatry Conference, Hawaii, October 2001, pp. 5 – 6.

Valley, P. (2004). Harold Shipman. The Independent, Wednesday 14th of January, Page 12.

Vallone, D., Picetti, R., Borelli, E. (2000). Structure and function of dopamine receptors. *Neurosci Biobehav Review*, 24, 125 – 132.

Van Krevelen, A. D. (1962). Early infantile autism and Autistic Psychopathy. *Journal of Autism and Childhood Schizophrenia*, vol. 1, no. 1, 84 – 85.

Van Krevelen, A. D., Kuipers, C. (1962). The psychopathology of Autistic Psychopathy. *Acta Paedopsychiatricia*, vol. 29, 22 – 31.

Viamontes, G., Beitman, B., Viamontes, C., Viamontes, J. (2004). Chapter 2: Neural Circuits for Self-awareness. From Self Awareness Deficits in Psychiatric Patients: Neurobiology, Assessment, and Treatment. Edited by B. Beitman and J. Nair. W. W. Norton & Company, New York: 2004.

Viding, E. (2004). Annotation: Understanding the development of psychopathy. *Journal of Child Psychology Psychiatry*, 45, 8, 1329 – 1337.

Viding, E., Blair, J. R., Moffitt, T. E., Plomin, R. (2005). Evidence for substantial genetic risk for psychopathy in seven year olds. *Journal of Child Psychology Psychiatry*, 46, 592 – 597.

Vlakeslee, S. (2005). Clues to Autism's Histories, International Herard Tribune, February 10th, Page 10.

Volkmar, F. R., Klin, A. (2000). Diagnostic issues in Asperger's syndrome. In Volkmar F. R., Klin A., Sparrow S. (2000). Asperger's syndrome. Guildford Press, New York.

Von Krafft-Ebing, R. (1886). The Psychopathia Sexualis (Revised Edition, 1965). London: Pantheon.

Von Krafft-Ebing, R. (1965). Psychopathia Sexualis (Trans F. S. Klaf). Staples Press. London.

Wallace, M. (1986). The silent twins. Penguin: Harmondsworth.

Warren, J., Hazelwood, R., Dietz, P. (1996). The Sexual Sadistic Serial Killer. *Journal of Forensic Science*, 41, 6, 970 – 974.

Watts and Morgan (1994). Malignant Alienation: Dangers for patients who are hard to like. *British Journal of Psychiatry*, 164, 11 – 15.

Wegner, D. M. (2002). The Illusion of Conscious Will. MIT Press, Cambridge, M.A.

Weightman, J. (1992). A Minor Monster. Times Literary Supplement, May 1st, Page 5.

West, A. H., Hill, V. (1995). Out of the Shadows. Simon and Schuster:

Wickelgri, I. (2005). Autistic Brains out of Synch? *Science*, 308, 1856 – 1856.

Widger, T. A., Cadoret, R., Hare, R. D., Robus, L. (1996). DSM-IV Antisocial Personality Disorder Field Trial. *Journal of Abnormal Psychology*, 105: 3 – 16.

Widiger, R. (2006). Chapter 8: Psychopathy and DSM-IV Psychopathology. Chapter in Handbook of Psychopathy, Edited by C. J. Patrick, Guildford Press, New York, 2006.

Widiger, T. A., Rogers, J. H. (1989). Prevalence and comorbidity of personality disorders. *Psychiatric Annals*, 19: 132 – 136.
Wilson, C. (1971). The Casebook of Murder. Mayflower: London.
Wing, L. (1981). Asperger's syndrome – a clinical account. *Psychological Medicine*, vol. 11, 115 – 129.
Wing, L. (1986). Classification of Asperger's syndrome. *Journal of Autism and Developmental Disorders*, vol. 16, 513 – 515.
Wing, L. (1991). Asperger's syndrome and Kanner's autism. In U. Frith (ed.) Autism and Asperger's syndrome, Cambridge: Cambridge University Press.
Wing, L. (1991). The relationship between Asperger's syndrome and Kanner's autism. In U. Frith (ed.) Autism and Asperger's syndrome, Cambridge: Cambridge University Press.
Wing, L. (1996). The Autism Spectrum. London: Constable.
Wing, L. (1997). Syndromes of autism and atypical development. In Handbook of Autism and Pervasive Developmental Disorder. Edited by Volkmar F., Paul R., Klin A., Cohen D. J. (2005). John Wiley & Sons.
Wing, L. (1998). The history of Asperger's syndrome. In E. Schopler, G. Mesibov, and L. Kunce (Eds) Asperger's syndrome or High Functioning Autism? New York: Plenum Press.
Wing, L., Gould, J. (1979). Severe impairments of social interaction and associated abnormalities in children: Epidemiology and classification. *Journal of Autism and Childhood Schizophrenia*, 9, 11 – 29.
Winn, P. (2001). Dictionary of Biological Psychology. Brunner Routledge: Hove.
Wolf, L. (1980). The Life and Crimes of Gilles de Rais. Bluebeard. New York: Clarkson N. Potter.
Wolff, S. (1990). Diagnostic precision or a confusion of terms: The example of Schizoid Disorders of Childhood. *British Journal of Clinical and Social Psychiatry*, 7, 59 – 65.
Wolff, S. (1995). Loners: the Life Path of Unusual Children, London: Routledge.
Wolff, S. (1998). Schizoid Personality in childhood: Links with Asperger's syndrome, schizophrenia, spectrum disorders, and elective mutism. In Schopler E., Mesibov G., Kunce L. (1998). Asperger's syndrome or High Functioning Autism? Plenum Press: New York.
Wolff, S. (2001). Book review. *Journal of Child Psychology Psychiatry*, 42, 8, 1104.
Wolff, S., Barlow, A. (1979). Schizoid personality in childhood: A comparative study of schizoid, autistic and normal children. *Journal of Child Psychology and Psychiatry*, 19, 175 – 180.
Woodworth, M., Porter, S. (2002). In cold blood: Characteristics of criminal homicides as a function of psychopathy. *Journal of Abnormal Psychology*, 111, 436 – 445.
World Health Organisation (1992) International Classification of Diseases (10th Edition), Geneva, Switzerland: author.
Wulffen, E. (1910). Enzyklopadie de modernen Kriminalistik. Langenscheidt, Berlin.
Yang, Y., Raine, A., Todd, L., Bihrle, S., Lancasse, L., Colletti, P. (2005). Prefrontal white matter in pathological liars. *British Journal of Psychiatry*, 187, 320 – 325.
Zimmer, C. (2005). The Neurobiology of Self. *Scientific American*, November, 65 – 71.

INDEX

A

abdomen, 87, 145
abnormalities, 3, 24, 43, 44, 57, 59, 60, 61, 62, 65, 76, 77, 78, 119, 188, 196
abusive, 148
ACC, 56, 57
accidental, 109
accommodation, 139
achievement, 131
acid, 141, 174, 193
activation, 49, 57, 61, 62, 64, 73, 96
acute, 10, 111, 149
adaptation, 47, 50, 57
addiction, 73, 126, 151
adjustment, 124
administration, 76
adolescents, 26, 38, 49, 63, 96, 117, 120, 148, 163, 164, 183, 191
adult, 8, 14, 21, 22, 23, 26, 33, 36, 58, 63, 64, 65, 74, 76, 77, 89, 98, 106, 125, 126, 129, 137, 139, 148, 159, 164, 183, 187, 193
adulthood, 10, 79, 84, 96, 187, 194
aetiology, 18, 98, 175, 176
affective experience, 47, 48
affective states, 79
age, 8, 12, 20, 28, 34, 45, 59, 63, 84, 85, 88, 93, 102, 106, 108, 121, 124, 127, 129, 135, 137, 143, 144, 148, 161, 163, 169, 190
agent, 48, 69, 88
aggression, 2, 19, 23, 33, 34, 35, 36, 45, 60, 61, 63, 65, 74, 75, 76, 77, 78, 79, 80, 84, 86, 94, 95, 123, 165
aid, 104, 108, 152

alcohol, 28, 35, 104, 118, 124, 135, 148, 153, 167, 191
alcohol consumption, 135
alcoholics, 112, 115
alienation, 37, 184
allele, 18, 55, 183
alternative, 42, 52, 116, 151, 174
altruism, 60
ambivalent, 109
American Indian, 192
American Psychiatric Association (APA), 8, 10, 14, 19, 20, 22, 26, 27, 99, 170, 175, 179
amino acid, 174
amputation, 87
amygdala, 18, 45, 59, 60, 61, 62, 63, 64, 66, 67, 68, 76, 95, 96, 98, 119, 165, 173
androgens, 78, 79
androgyny, 44, 134
anger, 25, 49, 61, 84, 87, 103, 110, 121, 135, 143, 170
animals, 11, 19, 60, 61, 78, 85, 88, 94, 106, 115, 124, 125, 133, 135, 136, 137, 144, 145, 166, 167, 168
anterior cingulate cortex, 61, 135
antimony, 107, 108, 137
antisocial acts, 34
antisocial behaviour, 16, 19, 22, 23, 29, 34, 49, 63, 74, 77, 180
antisocial personality, 20, 76, 154
antisocial personality disorder, 20
anus, 90
anxiety, 17, 24, 48, 50, 51, 77, 95, 110, 119, 172, 176
anxiety disorder, 17
aphasia, 29
apparel, 101
appetite, 2, 80, 159
application, 41
argument, 72, 166

arousal, 22, 45, 51, 60, 75, 79, 84, 85, 86, 92, 192
arrest, 108, 109, 157
arsenic, 159, 160, 161
arson, 34, 36, 37, 56, 122, 135, 166, 167
artistic, 104, 135
asphyxia, 109
assault, 34, 35, 36, 87, 119, 140
assessment, 35, 64, 180, 186
astronomy, 133
asymmetry, 30, 186
atmosphere, 132
atrocities, 127
attachment, 78, 79, 80, 84, 90, 104, 111
attacks, 37, 111, 119, 135, 137
attempted murder, 37
Attention Deficit Hyperactivity Disorder (ADHD), ii, iv, 14, 18, 26, 27, 28, 49, 53, 63, 64, 66, 74, 75, 130, 163, 183, 184, 187, 188, 189
attitudes, 44, 49, 65
attribution, 173, 175
authority, 72, 116, 122, 151, 153
Autistic Spectrum Disorders (ASD), 12, 49, 60, 63, 76, 77
autobiographical memory, 25, 42, 60
autoimmune, 115
automatic processes, 42
autonomic activity, 46
Autonomic Nervous System, 65, 66, 170
autopsy, 118
aversion, 85
avoidance, 10, 46, 50, 51, 78, 95
awareness, 26, 38, 41, 46, 47, 51, 60, 64, 69, 180, 195

B

babies, 2, 127, 162
BAS, 52
BDNF, 78
Behavioural Inhibition System (BIS), 50, 52
behaviours, 16, 46, 73, 77, 78, 79, 129
beliefs, 25, 69, 92, 148, 173, 176, 179, 182
bible, 83, 103, 117, 167
bile, 150
binding, 76, 77
biochemistry, 99
biological processes, 69
bipolar, 56
bipolar cells, 56
birth, 28, 56, 59, 172
birth weight, 172
black market, 139
blame, 11, 24, 42, 48, 90, 101, 111, 133

bleeding, 127
blind spot, 14, 89
blood, 33, 66, 76, 90, 91, 99, 105, 124, 125, 126, 144, 145, 146, 156, 157, 158, 168, 176, 196
blood flow, 176
body language, 38
body size, 56
body weight, 117
bomb, 117
bonding, 79, 113, 177
borderline, 10, 18, 44
Borderline Personality Disorder, 10, 18, 44, 170, 184, 193
boredom, 18, 24, 51
boys, 14, 23, 38, 46, 49, 63, 78, 89, 95, 96, 105, 115, 124, 127, 128, 130, 143, 181, 182
brain activity, 65
brain damage, 28, 61, 122
brain development, 77, 96
brain functioning, 97
brain growth, 59
brain size, 56, 59, 95
brain structure, 60, 70, 98, 173
breathing, 91
broad spectrum, 15
brutality, 28
bullying, 38
burglary, 125
burn, 67, 130, 157

C

cancer, 149
caregivers, 189
cast, 130
catatonic, 7
catecholamine, 77
category a, 4
catholic, 92
catholic church, 92
caucasian, 189
cell, 55, 56, 59, 77, 126, 177
cell death, 77
cerebellum, 59
cerebral asymmetry, 30, 186
cerebral cortex, 63, 67, 96, 171, 175
cerebral function, 171
cerebral hemisphere, 30, 67
cerebrum, 67, 95
charm, 15, 89, 108, 117, 120, 142
chemicals, 34
child abuse, 105, 139
childbirth, 66

Index

childhood, 1, 6, 7, 10, 14, 16, 19, 22, 23, 25, 68, 89, 95, 96, 97, 101, 115, 121, 122, 124, 135, 144, 145, 147, 152, 154, 164, 168, 190, 196
christians, 158
chromosome, 67
chronic stress, 66, 165
cingulated, 179
civil servant, 1
classification, 9, 182, 196
clients, 8
clinical symptoms, 60
clinically significant, 7, 8, 170
clinician, 26, 37, 193
close relationships, 10, 112
clubbing, 152
codes, 130
cognition, 60, 61, 63, 179
cognitive ability, 98
cognitive deficit, 52, 183
cognitive development, 7, 48, 181
cognitive domains, 57
cognitive flexibility, 53
cognitive function, 56, 62
cognitive performance, 67
cognitive process, 30, 170, 174
cognitive tasks, 67
coherence, 14, 17, 47, 121
coitus, 126
commissure, 67
communication, 3, 4, 8, 22, 23, 30, 44, 47, 58, 67, 68, 77, 107, 113
communism, 132
community, 1, 14, 97, 123, 138, 151
comorbidity, 26, 196
compassion, 152, 158
compensation, 92
competence, 35
complement, 56
complexity, 4, 43, 64, 120
complications, vi, 28
components, 30, 51
comprehension, 2, 104
concealment, 115
concentration, 58, 94
conception, 47, 187
concordance, 86
concrete, 25, 38, 41, 43, 44, 47, 49, 133, 169
conditioning, 15, 46, 50, 51, 60, 62, 63
Conduct Disorder, 14, 19, 26, 27, 49, 75, 77, 122, 163, 182, 186
conduct problems, 22, 77, 95, 163, 187
confession, 37, 114, 140, 141, 166, 167
confidence, 105

confinement, 147, 148
conflict, 16, 76
confusion, 21, 43, 44, 52, 196
conjecture, 131
connectivity, 42, 55, 56, 57, 59, 67, 95, 96, 165
consciousness, 44, 62, 72, 103, 118, 152, 154
conspiracy, 112, 134
conspiracy theory, 112
consumption, 92, 135
control, 10, 12, 16, 22, 25, 36, 43, 48, 51, 53, 60, 65, 69, 85, 86, 90, 91, 92, 99, 102, 103, 109, 110, 111, 113, 117, 119, 123, 124, 129, 132, 133, 135, 137, 139, 145, 150, 152, 153, 154
conversion, 103
corporal punishment, 130
corpus callosum, 58, 59, 67, 95, 171
correlation, 64
cortex, 4, 18, 29, 42, 43, 44, 56, 57, 58, 59, 60, 61, 62, 63, 64, 67, 68, 73, 74, 80, 96, 98, 135, 171, 175, 177, 179, 190
cortisol, 77, 78, 95
counsel, 140
courts, 74
creative process, 131
crimes, 2, 13, 23, 29, 34, 35, 36, 37, 70, 86, 87, 90, 91, 94, 97, 99, 103, 119, 125, 126, 127, 129, 132, 136, 137, 138, 140, 152, 160, 161, 164, 186
criminal activity, 16
criminal acts, 85, 89
criminal justice system, 69
criminal violence, 35
criminality, 23, 29, 34, 50, 51, 62, 171
criminals, 1, 14, 19, 23, 30, 37, 89, 97, 133, 158, 172
criticism, 29, 90, 129
cross-cultural, 190
CSF, 77, 193
cues, 22, 25, 26, 38, 45, 51, 52, 66
curiosity, 33, 47, 114, 138, 143
curriculum, 106, 166
cyanide, 34, 107

D

dangerousness, 86, 107, 108, 151, 188
death, 5, 24, 36, 77, 84, 90, 91, 92, 94, 108, 109, 110, 111, 112, 114, 115, 119, 123, 126, 127, 128, 129, 137, 138, 140, 141, 142, 148, 149, 150, 151, 152, 154, 156, 157, 158, 159, 161, 167, 186
death penalty, 110, 156
death sentence, 127
debt, 142
decision making, 60, 62, 68, 177
decisions, 4, 56, 62, 69

defects, 56
defence, 11, 33, 35, 99, 140, 142, 169
deficiency, 47, 53
deficits, 1, 6, 7, 15, 17, 20, 21, 24, 28, 33, 37, 42, 44, 46, 48, 49, 50, 51, 52, 53, 56, 57, 60, 63, 74, 75, 76, 89, 98, 109, 142, 150, 153, 163, 164, 183, 184, 192
definition, 4, 83, 117
degenerate, 87
degradation, 48, 74, 87, 91, 92, 103
delinquency, 74, 125, 188
delirium, 88
delusional thinking, 156
delusions, iii, 26, 37, 139, 156, 182
dementia, 127, 156
denial, 29
Department of Justice, 147, 148
depression, 17, 76, 92, 94, 104, 108, 110, 115, 119, 122, 133, 136, 140, 148, 151, 176
deprivation, 16
Desert Storm, 156
destruction, 72, 130, 136
detachment, 9, 10, 23, 24, 175
detection, 34, 45, 46
developmental delay, 52
developmental disorder, 9, 10, 52, 99, 171, 189
deviant behaviour, 69, 86
deviation, 110
Diagnostic and Statistical Manual of Mental Disorders, 179
diagnostic criteria, 3, 19
diarrhoea, 138
diet, 128
differential diagnosis, 5, 10, 23, 184
differentiation, 5, 8, 43, 77, 98, 188
diffusion, 10, 18, 44, 60, 65, 67, 85, 87, 102, 107, 110, 116, 118, 120, 130, 132, 134, 135, 138, 139, 140, 142, 150, 152, 154, 155, 166
dimorphism, 95
disability, 5, 8, 12, 19, 29, 35, 58, 70, 94, 99, 188, 193
discipline, 72, 112, 152
discomfort, 10, 48
discourse, 134
discrimination, 57
dishonesty, 49
disinhibition, 58
disorder, 3, 6, 7, 8, 9, 10, 14, 20, 22, 25, 26, 28, 29, 30, 36, 41, 45, 48, 52, 63, 74, 77, 78, 85, 99, 129, 164, 176, 187, 192, 193, 194, 195
disposition, 49, 74
distortions, 10, 11
distress, 24, 47, 50, 65, 66

diversity, 80
divorce, 79
DNA, 98
domestic violence, 101, 135
dominance, 19, 36, 86, 91
dopamine, 18, 21, 195
dopaminergic, 18
dosage, 67
DRD4 gene, 188, 189
drinking, 155
drowning, 120, 124
drug abuse, 28, 151
drug addict, 73, 149, 151
drugs, 35, 43, 163
DSM, 8, 9, 10, 14, 19, 20, 21, 22, 26, 27, 36, 195
DSM-II, 10, 14, 19
DSM-III, 10, 19
DSM-IV, 8, 9, 10, 19, 20, 21, 22, 26, 27, 36, 195
duration, 83

E

Eastern Europe, 42
eating, 90
ego, 20, 131, 134
ejaculation, 126, 145
elderly, 80, 149
electric charge, 119
elementary school, 115
embryo, 98
emission, 195
emotional experience, 20, 30, 61, 63, 175
emotional information, 43
emotional intelligence, 4, 185
emotional memory, 62, 169
emotional reactions, 22
emotional stimuli, 62
emotions, 4, 16, 17, 19, 25, 41, 42, 46, 47, 48, 49, 51, 57, 61, 62, 63, 65, 69, 88, 95, 109, 117, 152, 155, 169, 179, 189
employment, 110
engagement, 44, 75, 79, 153
enlargement, 64, 96
enterprise, 84
environment, 10, 14, 16, 28, 43, 63, 69, 71, 75, 120, 124
environmental factors, 14, 15, 17
environmental stimuli, 48
ethics, 72, 187
Europe, 88
evil, 22, 29, 44, 71, 72, 83, 97, 99, 104, 112, 117, 119, 120, 122, 130, 131, 135, 142, 144
evolution, 60, 66, 72, 179

excitability, 76
excuse, 34, 35, 118
execution, 80, 123, 126, 145, 154
executive function, 53, 60, 63
exercise, 129, 148
explicit knowledge, 52
exposure, 75, 79, 84, 87, 191
extinction, 121
eye contact, 78, 89, 170

F

face recognition, 56, 172
facial expression, 6, 46, 57, 76
factor analysis, 22
failure, 4, 13, 17, 19, 20, 21, 24, 50, 68, 85, 86, 112, 172
faith, 72
family, 5, 16, 68, 94, 102, 104, 106, 111, 112, 129, 134, 135, 137, 156, 163, 183
family environment, 16
family history, 111
family life, 134
family members, 94
FAS, 172
fat, 106
FBI, 83, 84, 86, 149
fear, 15, 20, 21, 36, 45, 46, 51, 60, 61, 62, 63, 64, 76, 77, 89, 92, 123, 130, 152, 169, 181
feedback, 86
feelings, 4, 10, 24, 25, 30, 43, 48, 49, 62, 64, 65, 68, 71, 77, 79, 88, 90, 92, 125, 128, 134, 154, 169, 170, 175, 177
females, 14, 66, 67, 68, 77, 79, 91, 94, 95, 110, 120, 146, 152, 157, 165, 166
fever, 148
film, 28, 50, 68, 155
fire, 35, 37, 68, 105, 106, 124, 147, 157
flatulence, 129
flexibility, 53
floating, 25, 116
flow, 33, 176
fMRI, 29, 57, 64
food, 3, 81, 101, 104, 122
forensic, 36, 64, 72, 191
forensic patients, 64
forensic settings, 191
forgiveness, 119
fragmentation, 11
fraud, 135, 136
free will, 43, 69, 98
freedom, 98, 130, 131, 132
freedom of choice, 98

friendship, 14, 89, 112
frontal cortex, 18, 59, 60, 61, 80, 135, 190
frontal lobe, 43, 44, 53, 58, 60, 61, 63, 72, 144, 172
frustration, 13, 15, 50, 134
functional imaging, 175
fusiform, 21, 57, 191
fusion, 84

G

GABA, 172
games, 41, 115, 131
Gamma, 172
gas, 37, 66, 111, 141
gender, 77, 88, 95, 105
gene expression, 78
general education, 124
general intelligence, 67
genes, 18, 27, 28, 59, 63, 67, 69, 71, 72, 78, 81, 85, 128, 151, 183, 188, 189
genetic abnormalities, 74
genetic factors, 15, 17, 28, 42, 51, 60, 67, 85, 175
genetic mutations, 72
genetics, 190
genocide, 72
genome, 163
genomics, 190
genotype, 17
gestation, 56
gifted, 104
girls, 23, 38, 88, 91, 102, 105, 124, 136, 137, 143, 144, 146, 157, 158
glucose, 21, 60, 67
glucose metabolism, 21, 60
goals, 63
god, 44, 60, 103, 121, 151
government, vi, 121, 155, 156
governors, 122
grain, 132, 160
grey matter, 21, 58, 59, 60
grief, 91, 136, 149
group therapy, 119
groups, 8, 26, 35, 38, 39, 53, 60, 81, 89, 113, 127, 141
growth, 59, 79, 95, 96
growth spurt, 59
guilt, 16, 17, 34, 45, 48, 57, 63, 102, 109, 111, 125, 135, 136, 137, 140, 145, 146, 152, 154, 155, 158, 159, 160, 172
guilt feelings, 154
guilty, 119, 123, 140, 155, 156
guns, 19, 155, 166
gyrus, 29, 57, 61, 64, 67, 68

H

handling, 136
hanging, 104, 134
happiness, 49
harbour, 86
harm, 18, 20, 46, 51, 71, 128, 135
hate, 61, 87, 121, 123
health, vi, 69, 163, 192
hearing, 111, 124
heart, 16, 33, 42, 75, 78, 95, 104, 109, 120, 144, 170
heart attack, 109
heart rate, 75, 78, 95, 170
heartbeat, 66, 105
helplessness, 164
hemisphere, 5, 30, 55, 57, 58, 66, 75, 79, 165, 183, 193
heredity, 20
heritability, 28
heterogeneity, 4, 11, 15, 21, 63, 64, 66, 102
hippocampal, 61, 64, 66, 165, 173
hippocampus, 18, 21, 59, 61, 66, 80, 98, 165, 173
homeless, 112
homicide, 84, 86, 87, 90, 92, 93, 96, 105, 192
homogenous, 20
homosexuality, 104, 112
homovanillic acid, 193
hopelessness, 164
hormone, 66, 78, 79, 80, 95, 165, 171
hospital, 36, 91, 120, 132, 149, 151, 186, 190
hostility, 25, 75, 79
human animal, 121
human brain, 55, 98, 182
human genome, 163
human nature, 124, 131, 132, 158
human values, 51, 87
humanity, 1
humiliation, 84, 92
humorous, 132
hunting, 80, 90, 104, 126
husband, 111, 133, 143, 151, 160
hygiene, 5
hyperactivity, 6, 7, 26
hypersensitive, 10, 11, 25, 38, 90, 106, 110, 129, 135
hypertensive, 66
hypertrophy, 4
hypothalamus, 60, 61, 173
hypothesis, 18, 29, 50, 56, 60, 65, 73, 74, 77, 86, 164

I

identical twins, 28
identity, 10, 18, 25, 44, 47, 49, 60, 62, 65, 67, 85, 87, 99, 102, 107, 116, 118, 120, 130, 132, 133, 134, 135, 138, 139, 140, 142, 150, 152, 153, 154, 155, 164, 170, 175, 189
identity diffusion, 10, 18, 60, 65, 67, 85, 87, 102, 107, 116, 118, 120, 130, 132, 134, 135, 138, 139, 140, 142, 150, 152, 154, 155
idiosyncratic, 37
illusion, 69, 128
images, 11, 53, 84, 107, 175, 188, 195
imagination, 2, 3, 47, 125, 127, 129, 141
imitation, 174
impairments, 3, 4, 37, 67, 190, 196
implants, 98
imprisonment, 109, 119, 125, 149, 159, 161
impulsive, 10, 14, 15, 16, 17, 19, 22, 50, 52, 60, 63, 74, 75, 76, 87, 111, 120, 129, 130, 134, 163, 170, 195
inactivation, 67
incarceration, 122, 153
incest, 130
incidence, 14
incurable, 121
independence, 22
indices, 78, 95
individual differences, 64, 192
infants, 59, 94, 161
infections, 115, 122, 167
inferences, 64
inferior frontal gyrus, 68
information processing, 42, 43, 52, 56, 191
inherited, 28, 29, 61
inhibition, 17, 45, 46, 50, 53, 60, 64, 73, 76, 135, 172, 188
injection, 149
injury, vi, 65, 87
injustice, 2, 125, 126, 137, 147
inmates, 107, 108, 158
insane, 123
insight, 5, 47, 49, 152, 153
instability, 10
instinct, 88, 135, 154
insults, 36, 129
insurance, 136
insurance companies, 136
integration, 29, 56, 58, 74, 95, 112
integrity, 60
intelligence, 3, 4, 29, 67, 101, 104, 110, 122, 124, 131, 145
intentions, 33
interaction, 4, 24, 28, 47, 50, 56, 57, 76, 87, 89, 114, 115, 116, 171, 176, 196
interference, 91

internal controls, 16
internalised, 16, 43
International Classification of Diseases, 127, 196
interpersonal communication, 3, 22
interpersonal contact, 102
interpersonal empathy, 37
interpersonal factors, 85
interpersonal relationships, 10, 22, 36, 56, 89, 170
interpersonal skills, 153
interview, 114, 189
intimacy, 112, 152, 153
intimidating, 19
introversion, 23, 24
introvert, 23
intuition, 57, 71
inventors, 11
Investigations, 98
iron, 128, 152, 157
irritability, 74, 75
isolation, 10, 24, 92, 104, 112, 128, 194

J

Jews, 1, 72, 107, 112, 113, 114
jobs, 136
judge, 44, 125, 127, 154
judiciary, 153
juries, 33, 153, 154
justice, 69, 133, 155, 187
justification, 127

L

lack of control, 135
language, 3, 4, 5, 7, 8, 20, 29, 30, 38, 41, 44, 46, 55, 56, 65, 67, 68, 79, 80, 95, 96, 110, 114, 131, 134, 153, 170, 177, 192
language development, 7, 41, 170
language processing, 30, 177
language skills, 95
later life, 1, 38
laterality, 79
laughter, 103
law, 34, 37, 38, 99, 104, 123, 125, 128, 129, 131, 132, 135, 136, 149, 152, 166
law enforcement, 38
learning, 6, 7, 12, 16, 42, 45, 46, 51, 58, 63, 68, 89, 148, 172, 173, 191, 192, 193
learning disabilities, 172, 192
left hemisphere, 5, 30, 66, 67, 79
lesions, 4, 60
libertarian, 182
liberty, 108, 156
libido, 173
life span, 29
lifestyle, 111, 136
lifetime, 113, 130
likelihood, 26, 85
limbic system, 59, 61, 65, 67, 69
limitation, 3
linguistic, 30, 46, 107, 134
linguistic processing, 30
linkage, 189
links, 57, 76
listening, 116
localised, 57, 95
location, 83
long-distance, 23
love, 11, 17, 52, 61, 105, 124, 160
lover, 91, 103, 155, 160
lying, 23, 49, 58, 91, 126, 154

M

magazines, 148
magnetic resonance spectroscopy, 190
magnetoencephalography, 67
maintenance, 56, 102
maladaptive, 53, 61, 63
males, 14, 66, 67, 68, 76, 77, 93, 94, 95, 120, 147, 156, 158, 160, 161, 165, 166
malicious, 25, 34
malignant, 27, 51
management, 46, 53, 66, 122, 132, 136
manipulation, 49
manure, 150
MAO, 74, 165, 174, 183
market, 139
marriage, 111, 136, 148, 156, 158
materialism, 131
mathematics, 48, 121, 129, 148, 166, 168, 170
maturation, 14
measures, 49, 53, 75, 95
media, 84, 91, 109
medial prefrontal cortex, 43, 61
median, 75
medical school, 151
medical student, 139, 167
medicine, 8, 163, 164
memory, 25, 42, 53, 60, 61, 62, 64, 66, 97, 102, 107, 112, 119, 124, 129, 148, 169, 173
men, 2, 18, 47, 66, 67, 72, 74, 75, 77, 80, 95, 97, 108, 112, 116, 118, 121, 122, 124, 155, 159, 160, 161, 165
mental disorder, 28, 98, 129

mental health, 69, 163
mental illness, 9, 28, 52, 98, 139, 187
mental processes, 51
mental representation, 68
mental state, 44, 48, 49, 57, 61, 119, 173
messages, 148
metabolic, 55, 67
metabolic rate, 67
metabolism, 21, 60
metabolite, 77, 173
migration, 56, 98
military, 79, 101, 156
minority, 34
mirror, 30, 41, 47, 68, 102, 135
mobility, 131
modality, 11
models, 55, 193
modulation, 60, 73, 189
modules, 173
modus operandi, 49, 88, 90
money, 124, 135, 151, 161
monks, 128
mood, 9, 17, 170, 174
mood disorder, 9
moral code, 13, 16
moral development, 183, 187
morality, 51, 71, 72, 128, 130, 181
morals, 72
morphine, 149
morphological, 64
mothers, 94, 109, 161, 163
motivation, 17, 37, 61, 64, 86, 115
motives, 34, 84, 92
motor coordination, 172
movement, 11, 68, 170
MRI, 59, 63
multidimensional, 43
murder, 1, 2, 16, 34, 37, 43, 83, 84, 85, 86, 87, 89, 91, 92, 94, 99, 104, 105, 106, 107, 114, 115, 116, 119, 120, 122, 126, 127, 128, 131, 138, 139, 143, 144, 145, 146, 152, 153, 154, 158, 188
mutations, 72, 74
myelin, 177

N

narcissistic, 10, 25, 44, 51, 71, 72, 79, 87, 90, 104, 107, 110, 112, 120, 124, 125, 127, 129, 132, 133, 137, 138, 141, 147, 150, 152, 153, 154, 155, 160, 174
nation, 112, 114
natural, 14, 89, 103, 131, 138
needles, 146

nefarious, 94
negative emotions, 48
negative experiences, 63
neglect, 16, 28, 42
nerve, 59, 63, 95, 171, 174, 176, 177
nerve cells, 59, 63, 95, 174, 176, 177
nervous system, 21, 55, 65, 66, 75, 170, 174
neural connection, 42, 56, 59
neural development, 77
neural networks, 57, 176
neural systems, 46, 60
neurobiological, 4, 9, 17, 66, 69, 164, 185
neurochemistry, 76
neuroimaging, 66, 164, 195
neuroleptics, 163
neurological disease, 192
neurons, 21, 42, 47, 55, 58, 59, 60, 63, 67, 68, 73, 74, 80, 96, 98, 165
neuropsychiatric disorders, 193
neuropsychiatry, 185
neuroscientists, 69
neurotic, 16
neurotransmitter, 75, 76, 171, 172, 176, 177
neurotrophic factors, 78
noise, 11, 37, 56, 110, 134
non-human, 60, 92
non-human primates, 60
normal, 1, 2, 9, 15, 20, 22, 23, 30, 42, 43, 45, 49, 55, 56, 58, 64, 65, 68, 70, 71, 72, 77, 78, 85, 87, 96, 98, 102, 104, 112, 116, 119, 126, 134, 138, 144, 153, 165, 168, 196
normal children, 196
normal development, 78
novel stimuli, 58
novelty, 18, 28, 74, 104, 109, 120, 126, 130, 133, 138, 141, 146, 151, 152, 163, 175, 188
novelty seeking, 18, 28, 74, 109, 120, 133, 141, 146, 151, 163, 188
nucleus, 50, 61, 63, 67, 73
nucleus accumbens, 73
nurses, 94, 107, 108

O

obedience, 113
objectification, 131
observations, 96
occipital lobe, 58
occupational, 7
oculomotor, 179
Oedipus, 24, 129
Oedipus complex, 24, 129

offenders, 21, 23, 24, 35, 36, 52, 64, 76, 78, 86, 97, 98, 189, 193
olfactory, 61, 173
openness, 34, 47
opium, 136
opposition, 160
Oppositional Defiant Disorder, 121, 122, 188
oral, 80
organ, 55, 139, 152, 163
organised crime, 86
organism, 73
orgasm, 88, 109, 118, 124, 126, 170
orientation, 44, 47
originality, 5
overload, 11, 111
oxytocin, 78, 79

P

paedophilia, 65, 131, 132
pain, 62, 65, 68, 85, 87, 109, 141, 143, 149, 155, 167, 168, 169, 173
panic attack, 119
paralysis, 144
paranoia, 156
parasympathetic, 170
parents, 12, 14, 23, 62, 89, 101, 105, 127
parietal, 175
parietal lobe, 57, 68
parole, 147
passive, 50, 75, 78, 95
pathology, 59, 68
pathways, 56, 58, 62
patients, 8, 9, 22, 23, 25, 27, 33, 36, 37, 50, 53, 55, 56, 61, 64, 65, 128, 131, 149, 151, 164, 168, 182, 195
peer, 5, 6, 35, 38, 89, 106, 140, 148, 170
peer group, 89
peer relationship, 5, 6, 148, 170
penalty, 110, 156
penis, 109, 119, 128
pensioners, 149
perception, 11, 37, 43, 61, 63, 67, 79
perfectionism, 10
personal relations, 94, 112, 153
personality disorder, vi, 8, 9, 10, 14, 15, 20, 44, 78, 85, 92, 99, 180, 187, 193, 196
personality traits, 17, 24, 28
personality type, 133
persuasion, 63, 157
PET, 175
pets, 106, 138
pharmaceutical, 109

pharmacological, 97
pharmacological treatment, 97
phenocopy, 24
phenomenology, 179
phenotype, 9, 17
phenotypic, 23
philosophers, 158
philosophy, 98, 122, 123, 128, 131, 132
photographs, 90, 109, 110, 125
phylogenetic, 55
physical world, 72
physiological, 45, 70
physiological arousal, 45
planning, 38, 53, 58, 60, 90, 94, 126, 141, 172, 176
plasma, 78
platelet, 76
play, 3, 51, 60, 62, 66, 67, 68, 78, 84, 85, 86, 96, 104, 120, 131, 150, 153
pleasure, 2, 19, 24, 62, 79, 85, 86, 88, 89, 92, 94, 109, 126, 127, 128, 129, 141, 145, 147, 151, 152, 159, 160, 166, 174
poisoning, 11, 34, 35, 37, 94, 106, 107, 108, 121, 122, 126, 129, 136, 137, 161, 162, 166
police, 38, 85, 90, 101, 102, 106, 107, 109, 110, 114, 119, 120, 126, 132, 137, 147, 152, 153, 166, 168
politicians, 2, 13
politics, 16, 81
pollution, 92
polymorphisms, 18, 21, 74, 151, 188
poor relationships, 123
population, 11, 12, 23, 25, 28, 34, 35, 36, 84, 192
Post Traumatic Stress Disorder, ii, iii, 17, 135
power, 1, 12, 52, 53, 55, 85, 86, 90, 92, 109, 113, 115, 117, 128, 133, 151, 154
pragmatic, 6, 7, 20, 29, 41, 44, 47, 117, 134, 170
precocious puberty, 78
predators, 71, 80, 97
prediction, 12, 17, 28
predisposing factors, 34
preference, 88, 91, 92
prefrontal cortex, 42, 43, 59, 61, 62, 67, 98
pregnant, 28, 101, 127, 138, 143, 155, 158, 172
pregnant women, 127, 158
preschool, 109
prevention, 164
prisoners, 27, 39, 99, 122, 123, 126, 148, 158, 159
prisons, 14, 89, 122, 132, 147, 149
private, 86, 128, 156
probands, 28
problem solving, 89, 175
processing deficits, 46, 50, 52
procreation, 128
production, 20, 29

profit, 94, 136, 161
prognosis, 100, 108
prolactin, 76, 191
promoter region, 189
property, vi, 88, 147
propranolol, 66
protection, 12, 68, 97
provocation, 75
proxy, 94
Prozac, 176
pruning, 59
pseudo, 102, 138, 153
psyche, 128, 134
psychiatric diagnosis, 133
psychiatric disorder, 66
psychiatrists, 9, 28, 103, 123, 128, 129, 133, 153
psychoanalysis, 188, 191
psychological functions, 27, 41
psychologist, 72, 111, 133, 152, 154
psychology, vi, 50, 104, 153
psychopathic, 2, 13, 14, 15, 16, 17, 18, 22, 23, 24, 25, 27, 28, 29, 37, 45, 46, 47, 49, 51, 60, 76, 77, 80, 81, 85, 89, 91, 95, 97, 99, 120, 127, 149, 176, 180, 181, 189, 190
psychopathic offenders, 97, 189
psychopathology, 10, 19, 114, 163, 164, 195
psychopaths, 16, 17, 18, 20, 22, 23, 28, 29, 30, 50, 51, 52, 61, 64, 65, 66, 97, 181, 185, 188, 190
psychosis, 26, 37, 137, 187
psychotherapy, 30, 97
psychotic, 37, 52, 85, 92
puberty, 78, 86, 109, 144
public, 1, 34, 72, 111, 125, 130, 150
publishers, 131
punishment, 45, 46, 50, 51, 56, 62, 76, 80, 88, 97, 122, 130
punitive, 122
Purkinje cells, 59

Q

questioning, 11

R

race, 113, 121, 123, 125, 126, 132
racism, 147
radar, 133
radiation, 108
random, 36, 102, 108, 134
range, 9, 10, 67, 84, 95, 96, 165
rape, 36, 86, 87, 109, 110, 128

reactivity, 22, 64, 66, 75, 77, 78, 95, 176
reading, 5, 26, 38, 48, 63, 68, 110, 112, 122, 131, 163, 165, 167, 170
reading skills, 163
reality, 3, 8, 24, 35, 41, 105, 120, 127, 129, 131, 134, 135, 154, 156
reasoning, 30
recall, 66, 148
receptors, 57, 195
recidivism, 14, 17, 29, 97
reciprocity, 6, 46, 48, 112, 167, 170
recognition, 41, 47, 48, 56, 63, 76, 172, 181
recovery, 108
recreational, 84
rectum, 146
recurrence, 86
reflexes, 71
refuge, 105, 112
regional, 56, 77, 96
regular, 90, 106
regulation, 25, 47, 61, 76, 91, 174, 183, 193
rehabilitation, 108, 163
rejection, 1, 25, 34, 89, 90, 92, 118, 134, 135
relevance, 29, 30, 56, 158
religion, 72, 92, 130
religious beliefs, 92
rent, 102
resources, 30
responsiveness, 17, 75
retaliation, 156
retention, 3, 56
rewards, 18
right hemisphere, 5, 57, 58, 66, 75, 79, 165, 183
rigidity, 23
risk, 16, 18, 20, 21, 25, 26, 27, 41, 50, 55, 63, 73, 74, 75, 81, 86, 133, 152, 182, 183, 188, 195
robberies, 36, 121
robotic, 42, 51, 56, 115
routines, 4, 6, 35
Russian, 154, 161

S

sacred, 154
sadism, 84, 87, 88, 91, 126, 127, 158, 168, 169
sadness, 45, 49
safety, 19, 20, 21
satisfaction, 2, 15, 51, 87, 94, 110, 124, 125, 126, 134, 138
schizophrenia, 6, 7, 9, 25, 26, 37, 43, 71, 85, 92, 102, 110, 117, 156, 182, 187, 192, 195, 196
Schizotypal Personality Disorder, 10, 23, 176

school, 5, 34, 38, 68, 101, 106, 111, 115, 116, 122, 124, 129, 130, 133, 142, 147, 148, 149, 151, 152, 163, 166, 167, 168, 183
school performance, 106, 166, 167, 168
scores, 26
scrotum, 146
search, 105
secret, 83, 94
security, 36, 149
self, vii, 41, 47, 131, 180, 187, 194, 195, 196
self image, 10
self representation, 41, 43
self-awareness, 26, 41, 60, 64, 180
self-care, 138
self-concept, 51
self-consciousness, 44
self-destruction, 130
self-esteem, 25, 89, 91, 92, 102, 120, 154, 176
self-help, 7
self-image, 10
self-interest, 51
self-observation, 41
self-recognition, 41
self-report, 49, 86
semantic, 20, 29, 30, 41, 47, 117, 134, 186
semantic processing, 29, 186
semen, 146
sensation, 3, 24, 28, 46, 47, 62, 74, 75, 77, 88, 104, 109, 120, 130, 138, 145, 163
sensation seeking, 28, 46, 74, 75, 77, 109, 130, 163
sensitivity, 22, 23, 24, 38, 45, 62, 66, 77, 141, 143
sensory modality, 11
sentences, 38, 153
separation, 62, 160
serial murder, 66, 83, 84, 85, 86, 88, 93, 120, 141
series, 4, 20, 37, 46, 75
severity, 4, 8, 19, 26, 36, 60
sex, 65, 66, 67, 78, 79, 84, 85, 88, 92, 95, 96, 101, 102, 103, 118, 125, 127, 128, 130, 135, 140, 145, 159, 160
sex differences, 66, 67, 95
sex hormones, 66
sexual abuse, 16, 17, 28, 124, 131
sexual activity, 87, 90, 92, 112, 130
sexual assault, 2, 102, 119, 120, 140
sexual behaviour, 34, 102
sexual contact, 80
sexual deviancy, 61
sexual dimorphism, 95
sexual identity, 87, 107, 116, 130, 139
sexual intercourse, 124, 126, 145
sexual offences, 34, 35, 37
sexual violence, 86

sexuality, 84, 144
sexually abused, 122, 124, 139, 144, 145, 154
shame, 13, 20, 21, 24, 37, 50, 71, 119, 146, 172
sharing, 14, 30
shoot, 158
short period, 114
shortage, 81
shy, 23, 89, 92, 106, 109, 115, 137, 139, 144, 146, 152, 153, 156, 167
siblings, 88, 135
signals, 11, 62, 73
signs, 37, 86, 140
sites, 67, 98
skills, 4, 7, 23, 30, 38, 41, 62, 66, 67, 68, 89, 95, 110, 122, 129, 132, 135, 142, 148, 153, 155, 163, 168, 170
skin, 78, 95, 103, 115, 134, 158, 159
skin conductance, 78, 95
slaves, 101
smoking, 75, 188
SNP, 189
social activities, 26
social behaviour, 34, 51, 57, 60, 68
social cognition, 60, 61, 63
social context, 85
social distance, 38
social environment, 43, 120
social factors, 16
social impairment, 37, 190
social integration, 112
social isolation, 10, 24, 112, 194
social justice, 133
social learning, 42, 89
social life, 48, 118
social maladjustment, 37
social norms, 17, 19, 20, 21, 46, 74
social order, 43
social relations, 3, 9, 10, 24, 25, 26, 36, 38, 56, 57, 58, 89, 103, 107, 110, 112, 116, 122, 129, 133, 134, 139, 150, 151, 166, 168
social situations, 44, 56, 153
social skills, 38, 41, 110, 148, 170
social structure, 50
social withdrawal, 10
socialisation, 22, 36, 60, 63, 74, 131
socio-emotional, 5, 15, 60
sociology, 15, 158
sociopath, 14, 15, 16, 135
sodomy, 121, 122, 129, 130
solitude, 145
somatization, 25
somatization disorder, 25
sounds, 3, 156

spatial, 79, 173, 175
spatial ability, 79
spatial processing, 175
special interests, 3, 23, 34
specialisation, 57, 79
species, 2, 56, 93, 95
SPECT, 76, 176
spectroscopy, 190
spectrum, 5, 12, 15, 19, 21, 23, 26, 27, 49, 78, 164, 196
speculation, 131
speech, 3, 5, 7, 8, 30, 65, 114, 176
sperm, 155
spheres, 104
spontaneity, 5
sports, 115
stages, 90, 130, 136
statutes, 99
stem cells, 98
stereotypes, 110
stimulus, 18, 51, 62, 163
stock, 101
strategies, 64, 153, 163
strength, 83, 92, 120
stress, 10, 51, 66, 75, 165
stressors, 66
striatum, 61, 64, 174
students, 106, 149, 183
subgroups, 36, 75, 78
subjective, 47, 64
substance abuse, 79
substances, 169, 177
substitutes, 12, 164
suffering, 19, 28, 30, 72, 84, 92, 115, 156
suicide, 25, 75, 92, 106, 110, 112, 113, 119, 123, 124, 139, 141, 149, 151
superego, 20, 63, 109, 119, 133, 147, 148, 156
superiority, 26
survival, 81
suspects, 44
sympathetic, 5, 47, 62, 66, 71, 75, 170, 174
sympathetic nervous system, 75, 174
symptoms, 16, 17, 26, 29, 60, 64, 66, 74, 77, 78, 92, 108, 134
synapses, 28, 174, 176
synchronization, 58
synthesis, 43
systems, 46, 52, 59, 60, 69, 75, 170

T

talent, 55, 136, 148
targets, 93, 151

teachers, 122
teaching, 71
teens, 11
temperament, 23, 45, 75, 104, 182
temporal, 29, 57, 61, 64, 65, 67, 68, 80, 144, 177
temporal lobe, 61, 65, 67, 177
tension, 30, 87, 110
terrorist, 128, 160
testosterone, 67, 69, 77, 78, 79, 95, 165, 169
testosterone levels, 78
thalamus, 61, 62
thallium, 108
theft, 103, 121, 128, 141
therapeutic community, 97
therapy, 62, 98, 116, 119
thinking, 3, 4, 8, 36, 41, 43, 47, 61, 86, 119, 120, 130, 134, 149, 156, 170, 171, 175, 176
threat, 17, 19, 46, 60, 83, 110, 124, 144
three-dimensional, 95
threshold, 155, 167, 168
throat, 126, 144, 157
tolerance, 15, 87
torture, 83, 86, 87, 120, 127, 128, 131, 137, 158
toxicology, 107
tracers, 176
tradition, 157
training, 101, 107, 151, 163
trait anxiety, 77, 95
traits, 1, 9, 14, 17, 19, 22, 24, 25, 28, 33, 51, 77, 78, 89, 95, 103, 107, 111, 129, 163, 180, 184
transfer, 79
translation, 9, 33
transmission, 183
transplantation, 98
trial, 75, 107, 109, 117, 120, 125, 126, 127, 137, 138, 140, 157
tribal, 92
trust, 57
twins, 28, 195
tyramine, 174

U

uncertainty, 56
unemployment, 37
uniform, 158
urine, 75, 146

V

vagina, 90
validity, 77, 95, 186

values, 17, 22, 51, 64, 80, 87, 89, 98, 128, 130, 132
variance, 9, 23, 51, 60, 63, 182
vasopressin, 57, 78, 79
vein, 105
verbal fluency, 53
videotape, 118
Vienna Circle, 116
violence, vi, 5, 8, 13, 14, 16, 17, 19, 20, 23, 24, 33, 34, 35, 36, 45, 49, 63, 64, 74, 75, 76, 77, 78, 84, 85, 86, 87, 89, 94, 97, 98, 101, 120, 126, 128, 135, 142, 180, 184, 195
violent behaviour, 195
violent offenders, 24, 64
violent recidivism, 17
viruses, 108
viscera, 87, 119, 120
visual area, 68
visual processing, 56
visual stimuli, 177
visuospatial, 5
voice, 23, 30, 71, 114, 117, 141, 150
voles, 177
volunteers, 186
vomiting, 66
vulnerability, 71
vulnerable people, 128, 137, 154

W

war, 80, 112, 113, 123, 128, 155
warfare, 81, 104
weakness, 127
weapons, 19, 81, 133
web, 55
West Africa, 122
white matter, 21, 58, 67, 95, 96, 196
witchcraft, 157
withdrawal, 3, 10, 45, 51, 133
wives, 161
women, 2, 23, 66, 67, 72, 73, 77, 80, 83, 84, 85, 87, 89, 92, 93, 94, 101, 102, 103, 109, 110, 113, 120, 126, 127, 134, 136, 137, 139, 140, 141, 142, 145, 146, 152, 154, 157, 158, 160, 167, 189
word processing, 29
workers, 110, 124, 161
Workers Party, 112
working memory, 53
World Health Organisation (WHO), 15, 196
World War, 112, 113, 114, 139, 140, 150
worry, 121
writing, 47, 88, 109, 130, 131, 132, 134, 166, 168

Y

young women, 146, 154, 157

Z

zinc, 160